Not Discussed

_ the unspoken rules for a career _
in academic medical research

Not Discussed

_ the unspoken rules for a career _
in academic medical research

C. Michael Stein

Not Discussed
– the unspoken rules for a career in academic medical research –

ISBN: 978-1-7216-2502-4

Cover design: C. Michael Stein
Page layout and pre-press: Lighthouse24

C. Michael Stein
2011 Sweetbriar Avenue
Nashville, TN 37212
cmichaelstein@gmail.com

Contents

Acknowledgments

Thanks to my mentors and mentees, past and present. Nothing in this book is new; I have tried to attribute ideas to their sources and apologize if I have forgotten the origin of some. Thanks to Cecilia Chung, Michelle Ormseth, Keisha Hardeman, Jorge Gamboa, and Josh Fessel for providing helpful suggestions. Also, thanks to the many organizations that support patients, research, and the careers of young investigators. Royalties from this edition will be donated to the Arthritis Foundation and the Lupus Research Alliance.

Introduction

This book is for people with an MD or PhD or similar degree who are starting or thinking of starting a research career in academic medicine. It focuses on the components of career development beyond your primary research and clinical work. You will not learn how to design a study or how to troubleshoot a Western blot. Rather, you will learn how to play the game of academic medicine with its arcane rules that are usually learned through bitter experience. When I began my career I thought that if I immersed myself in science everything else would take care of itself, and in an ideal world that would be the case. Until then, this book contains lessons I wish I had learnt earlier. The opinions expressed in the book are my own and should not be taken to reflect the opinions of any institution or funding agency. The book is a collection of personal observations (some of which may be wrong) not dogmatic advice – you can choose among many routes to reach your academic destination. Good luck.

Please email me if you spot typos, bad grammar, or errors. Suggestions about content are particularly welcome.

Thank you.

cmichaelstein@gmail.com

Chapter 1

What is a career in "academics"? – The different tracks

"I'm thinking about staying in academics"

Candidates who interview for postdoctoral fellowship positions often say, "I am thinking about staying in academics because I love to teach, and I think I would like to do some research, and I enjoy seeing patients." To plan an academic career you need to understand how these interests fit together.

A career in academic medicine requires income

An important question for your future career is how you will pay your salary. A medical school will negotiate a salary with you and that will involve a plan for you to generate income. Some medical schools provide some support for faculty, but at many you are responsible for generating most of your salary.

Generating your salary

There are two major ways to generate your salary: research grants and clinical practice. Teaching, the activity that attracts many to the academic world, is not usually a major source of salary. Other than a few people such as deans or directors of teaching programs, most academic medical faculty do not generate significant salary from teaching.

The triple threat – a rare species

Historically, academic physicians have aspired to excellence in research, clinical practice, and teaching – the so-called triple threat. Several evolutionary changes have made this a rare species. These changes include pressure to see more patients, decreased re-imbursement for clinical care, greater competition for grants, and increased administrative demands (1).

Efficient clinical practice is high-volume

Reimbursement for non-procedural specialties is low. This means that most physicians cannot support their research time through limited clinical practice. You cannot generate two days of salary from one day of clinical practice. In fact, it is challenging to generate one day of salary from one day of practice. Clinical medicine has evolved to be more efficient, and high-volume clinicians build systems to maximize efficiency. Thus they have an advantage over part-time, low-volume clinicians. Paradoxically, unexpected clinical demands are less disruptive for a full-time clinician because it is easier to accommodate an unexpected urgent visit if you have eight clinics a week than if you have one.

Efficient research is high-volume

Research has also evolved and competition for grants is fierce. Getting a grant is competitive, and review panels do not consider your clinical load. They decide based on scientific merit. Part-timers compete against full-timers. This is like an excellent amateur athlete competing against a professional. People who do research most of the time are more likely to obtain grant funding.

Clinical and research tracks in academic medicine

Several career tracks have evolved in response to the changing demands of clinical practice and research. Many medical schools appoint new faculty to a particular track. In that way, everyone knows what is expected. The five major tracks have different salary structures, responsibilities, expectations, and criteria for promotion and tenure (Chapter 20).

    1) The physician-scientist and tenure track investigator: This track is for physicians, and at some institutions, nurses, psychologists, pharmacists, and other health professionals who spend most of their time (~80%) doing research and are on the tenure track. They support themselves through NIH grants, initially K-awards and then RO1 grants, and their clinical work is limited – e.g., for MDs a half-day clinic once a week and a few weeks a year on the inpatient service. Their teaching responsibilities are also limited and are usually related to their particular area of research. Physician-scientists generate most of their salary through grant support and are judged by their publications, their ability to obtain grants, and their national and international scientific reputations.

    2) The clinician-scholar/clinician-educator: The terms clinician-scholar and clinician-educator are sometimes used interchangeably (CS or CE track) although they are different. People in this track spend most of their time (~80%) doing clinical work and the rest in scholarly activities that include research, writing review articles and book chapters, serving on national committees, and education. Clinician-scholars are the workhorses of academic medical centers. They are responsible for most of the patient care and teaching. Almost all clinician-scholars teach as part of their clinical work. However, some focus on medical education, and their track is sometimes designated the clinician-educator track. Clinician-educators often direct residency or fellowship training programs or have a research interest in teaching methods. They often have additional training in medical education. Clinician-scholars generate their salaries from patient care and are judged by the quality of the care they provide as well as their scholarly achievements. The quality and quantity of scholarly activities are important for promotion on the clinician-scholar track, but so too are teaching and clinical activities (Chapter 20). At many medical schools clinician-scholars are not eligible for tenure.

3) Medical center clinician: Medical center clinicians (MCCs) spend all their time on patient care. Bedside teaching is part of these activities, but MCCs are not expected to pursue scholarly activities.

4) Tenured or tenure-track scientist: This track includes PhD scientists who are principal investigators on NIH grants and direct, or plan to direct, their own research programs. Their teaching responsibilities are limited and are usually related to a particular area of research. Tenure-track scientists generate their salary through grants and are judged by their publications, their ability to obtain grants, and their national and international scientific reputations.

5) Non tenure-track scientists: These PhD scientists usually do not have their own large grants or research programs. Rather, they work with investigators who have NIH grants and contribute to the group's success. They seldom have teaching responsibilities and are judged by their publications, contributions to the success of large research programs, and national and international scientific reputations.

6) Other tracks: There are also several less well-defined tracks.

> ***The undifferentiated track:*** There is an unrecognized track – the undifferentiated young academic scientist. This track includes many people in the research years of a clinical fellowship or in a T32 postdoctoral fellowship. Many of these trainees do not have a definite career path but are interested in trying research. They use this time to make decisions about the future. *If you are an undifferentiated scientist, you must behave like a physician-scientist or tenure-track scientist during the early years of your research training.* In other words, you should choose a mentor and project as if it is for a long-term, research-intense career in science (Chapters 2 and 3), and spend as much time as possible doing research. People who devote 50 percent of their time to research with a weak mentor to see "if they take to research" find it difficult to establish a career if they decide later that research is what they want to do. On the other hand, someone who spends two or three years doing 90 percent research with an outstanding mentor can later decide against a research-intense career and easily move in another direction.

Administrative track: Most academic scientists in medical schools have minor administrative responsibilities, but some choose careers with larger roles. These career tracks can be in research and teaching (e.g., dean, associate dean, residency director), or in patient care (e.g., hospital administration).

Clinical trialist track: There are different types of clinical trialists. Some initiate their own trials, obtain NIH grants, and write papers about the work – their career can fall completely within the physician-scientist track. Others perform studies sponsored by industry, or are local investigators for multi-site trials. These studies are not primarily their own idea, and if they are published the local investigators are seldom the primary authors. This track is often a subtrack of the clinician-scholar track but is often flexible so that some people (provided there are enough trials to support their effort) spend much more than 20 percent of their time in research.

Other tracks: There are many hybrid tracks; you likely know people with academic careers that do not fall neatly into one of the tracks above. Institutions tend to be flexible about less orthodox career tracks if you can support yourself and the institution benefits from your career structure. People with an unorthodox career track often started on a more conventional one that evolved.

The five major career tracks in academic medicine					
	Physician-Scientist	Clinician -Scholar/ Educator	Medical Center Clinician	Tenure Track Scientist	Non-tenure Track Scientist
Clinical	20%	80%	100%	0%	0%
Research	80%	20% Research Education Scholarly activity	0%	100%	100%
PI of NIH grants	Yes	No	No	Yes	No
Tenure track	Yes	Not at most institutions	No	Yes	No
Primary yardsticks	Grants Papers Reputation	Clinical Scholarship Reputation	Clinical	Grants Papers Reputation	Papers Research team Reputation
Secondary yardsticks	Citizenship Clinical work Teaching	Citizenship	Citizenship	Citizenship Teaching	Citizenship

Summary

1 An academic medical career is defined by how you generate your salary.

2. Different career tracks have different expectations, tasks, and yardsticks.

3. People who spend most of their time doing research are more likely to be successful in the physician-scientist or tenure-track scientist pathways.

4. One size does not fit all; there are many different successful career tracks.

5. If you are in a trainee research position and are uncertain whether you want a long-term research career or not, behave as if you do.

Resources

1. Stein CM. Academic clinical research: Death by a thousand clicks. Sci Transl Med. 2015;7(318):318fs49. PMID: 26676604.

2. Tong CW, Ahmad T, Brittain EL et al. Challenges facing early career academic cardiologists. J Am Coll Cardiol 2014;63:2199-208. PMID:24703919

3. Coleman MM, Richard GV. Faculty career tracks at U.S. medical schools. Acad Med. 2011 Aug;86(8):932-7. PMID:21694565.

Chapter 2
Choosing your mentor

Look before you leap – choose your mentor carefully

One of the most important decisions you will make if you're planning a research career is choosing a mentor. Even if you're not planning a long-term research career, your choice of mentor will determine how successful your research time is. Your relationship with some mentors will be long-term, and if your career is successful, can be similar to a family relationship. You cannot pick your family, but you can pick your mentor. You would give a lot of thought to picking a guide for a three-year road trip, so why not give thought to picking your mentor? Thinking through the following steps will help.

1) Why are you looking for a research mentor?

People do research for many reasons; for example, to fulfill a program requirement, to buff up a CV and be more competitive for a fellowship, to try it out, and to be an academic scientist. All are valid reasons, but they embody different long-term aspirations and have different mentoring needs. The more committed you are to the possibility of a long-term career in academic research, the more important your choice of mentor.

2) What do you want from your research time?

Beginning researchers have many different goals; for example, to complete a project, to publish a paper, to get a sound training in the basics of research, to decide if research is a viable career path, and to build the foundation for a future scientific career. Different goals and career tracks (Chapter 1) need different preparation, mentors, projects, and commitment.

3) What do you want to do?

Before you look for a mentor, think about the research you want to do. Do you want to do bench research? Work with mice? Do clinical research with patients? Perform epidemiologic or genetic research in large datasets? Your personality and skills will influence your preferences, but keep an open mind and avoid rigid preconceptions. Starting research is an opportunity to explore new areas and learn new skills. Choose a broad research area that fascinates you, but remember that your initial training is a stepping stone – it is more important the stone be secure and well-trodden than that it fit your idealized preconceptions.

4) Looking

Look widely: It is daunting to look for a potential mentor outside your immediate circle, but don't be intimidated into a narrow search. Discuss possibilities with your research peers, particularly those who are a year or two ahead of you. Speak to a senior advisor in your division responsible for trainee development. Visit the websites of different departments and explore their faculty and research. Search faculty members in PubMed and see what they have published.

Finding a great mentor is more important than finding the ideal project: When you are searching for a mentor, it is best not to be rigidly committed to a preconceived project (Chapter 3). For example, you may want to study antioxidants in scleroderma lung disease and find that there is no one at your institution with a scleroderma research program. There may, however, be an antioxidant program in asthma that is ideal for your training. If your search is too narrow, you will discard possibilities that could provide an outstanding mentor and training. Much of the fundamental scientific training you get does not depend specifically on your project – it depends more on the mentor and the broad area of research. Once you have looked, thought, and discussed the options, make a list of potential mentors and then narrow the choice.

5) Narrowing the choice

How does one choose a mentor? People choose mentors for a range of different reasons – some good, some bad (Table).

Poor reasons for choosing a mentor	
Timing	Dr. X rounded with me first and suggested a project...
Admiration	Dr. X is a wonderful clinician and role model...
Subservience	The Chief of X offered me a project...
Familiarity	Dr. X was my chief resident...
Gullible	Dr. X was so enthusiastic...
Obligation	At the time I couldn't say no to Dr. X...
Spur of the moment	Dr. X and I saw a case and thought up an easy project...

Good reasons for choosing a mentor	
Success	Dr. X published 50 papers, has 2 RO1's and mentored...
Time	Dr. X makes time for trainees...
Expertise	Dr. X is internationally recognized in my research area...
Resources	Dr. X has the funding, equipment, and technicians I need...
Character	Dr. X is enthusiastic, supportive, fair and I like...
Clout	Dr. X has influence in my institution and nationally...

Different mentors suit different people. It is a mistake to automatically choose the mentor with the biggest lab, the most publications, or the most influence. To narrow your choice, weigh the mix of characteristics that follow.

Past success in science and mentoring: A strong mentor is experienced and has been successful in several areas – publishing papers, obtaining funding, *and* mentoring trainees. A PubMed search is important because it will tell you the breadth, quantity, and quality of your potential mentor's work. A RePORTER search will tell you about the mentor's NIH funding (1). Your mentor must have funding for you to do research. You should find out about the happiness and success of past trainees by speaking to people working in the lab and those who recently left. Fame and a large lab do not automatically make a good mentor. Ask lab members how often they meet with the mentor, how responsive the mentor is, if trainees go to national meetings, how much they publish, if they collaborate with each other, what they like, what they don't like, how collegial the lab is, and if anyone has been unhappy with the lab and what the problem was.

Your mentor's past success becomes your success: In addition to increasing your chances of success, there are other reasons to choose an established and successful mentor. When you apply for a K-award, the strength of your mentor is one of the criteria reviewers consider. If your mentor does not have a track record of success, your application (no matter how good) will struggle. Choose a K-quality mentor.

Most successful mentors are associate or full professors: Your mentor must have sustained, independent RO1 or equivalent funding if you plan to have a career in science. Therefore, most proven mentors will be associate or full professors. What happens if the person who inspires you most is an assistant professor with only a K-award? It would be poor grantsmanship and risky for your career to have this person as your primary mentor for a K application. What you can do is have a primary mentor who is a senior scientist and also a secondary mentor (or mentor-in-training) with whom you do most of your day-to-day work. Be careful. When your career trajectory and that of your mentor are only a few years apart, a potential problem is that you compete. This is less likely to happen if the mentor is senior and no longer fighting to establish independent success.

Time for you: There is little point in having a mentor who has no time for you. It is difficult to function with a mentor who can only schedule a 30 minute meeting if given a month's notice and then checks email throughout the meeting. Successful mentors are busy and often travel a lot. But somehow they seem to be available. Different mentors have different styles, and this affects how much time they spend with you. Some may supervise your activities very closely, "I'll see you at 8 a.m. and we can talk about what you are going to do today"; others may not, "Let's meet in a few weeks when you have completed these experiments and look at the data." Speak to other mentees to make sure that you understand the mentor's style.

Expertise, reputation, and resources: Your mentor must be a top-notch scientist. A mentor who has deep knowledge and good resources and is an outstanding scientist benefits you in many ways. First, your mentor will guide you to perform and interpret important experiments. Great scientists can identify important questions and approach them in ways that less talented scientists are not able to do. Second, your mentor will have a network of contacts that will be a source of advice and collaboration and will later provide reference letters for your promotion. Third, your mentor's resources become your resources. When you start research you have nothing – no bench, no pipette, and no money for an assay. You depend entirely on your mentor's resources. As you transition to independence, you need even more support, because most career-development grants provide your salary but do not provide enough money to perform the studies you described in your grant. It is tough to establish your research unless your mentor has resources and is committed to helping you.

Character, personality, and style: Consider the mentor's character, personality, and style. How would these affect you? Some mentors micro-manage like an anxious parent. They supervise every component of every experiment and can stifle your ability to think for yourself. Others are distant, more like a benign aunt or uncle that you see at Thanksgiving. Some mentors are socially adept, others are awkward. Some are tough on their mentees, others tell you that you can be anything you want to be. An excellent fit for one person may be the mentor from hell for another. There is no perfect mentor; your relationship will face challenges (Chapter 4). A mentor should be enthusiastic about science and about you. Some desirable and undesirable characteristics of a mentor are listed in the Table and discussed.

Perfect Mentor *	Imperfect Mentor
1. Teacher	1. Absentee landlord
2. Sponsor (Godfather, fixer)	2. Benevolent landlord
3. Advisor	3. Dictator
4. Agent (Lobbyist, advocate)	4. Self-promoter
5. Role Model	5. Jerk
6. Coach	6. Parent, judge, critic, taskmaster
7. Confidante	7. Gossip
8. Giver	8. Taker
9. Mind reader	9. Steamroller
10. Plays well with others	10. Throws toys
11. Able to let go	11. Hangs on
12. Observes boundaries	12. Poor boundary recognition
13. Can read a map	13. Wanders all over the place
14. Is not responsible for you	14. Is responsible for you

* The first seven characteristics of a perfect mentor are from an excellent article: Tobin MJ. Mentoring: seven roles and some specifics. Am J Respir Crit Care Med 2004;170: 14-117 (2).

Teacher vs. Absentee landlord: A good mentor, by spending time with you and your project, will teach you without seeming to do so. A mentor who is never around but is an author on your papers is more like an absentee landlord collecting the rent. Good mentoring exposes you to not only new scientific areas but also to new ways to think, talk, write, behave, and relate to the world.

Sponsor vs. Benevolent landlord: A mentor smoothes your path – this can be an introduction to another scientist, providing you with access to something you need, a quiet word in the ear of your division chief, and so on. A mentor who is not engaged but has provided you with space in which to work is a benevolent landlord rather than a mentor. Ensure that you and your mentor do not have different views of the relationship; someone you view as a mentor may view his or her role as that of a facilitator (i.e., you are someone "spending some time in the lab").

Advisor vs. Dictator: It is difficult for a mentor to give advice without seeming to dictate a particular path. A good mentor will help you evaluate options; a poor mentor will dictate the path. A good mentor also knows when it is important to lead towards a particular path. However, you are responsible for your path and your success.

Advocate vs. Self-promoter: A good mentor is on your side and advocates for you by promoting your strengths and achievements. Unfortunately, some mentors, even after achieving just about everything possible, are set on promoting themselves by taking advantage of their trainees' achievements.

Role model vs. Jerk: How your mentor behaves is important. Mentors who are honest, enthusiastic, generous, knowledgeable, reliable, and who have fire in the belly are people you trust and want to emulate. Ideally, your mentor would be a perfect role model for all aspects of life. That almost never happens – all mentors have quirks – but avoid those who lie, cheat, and shout, and those who are irrational, paranoid, racist, sexist, passive-aggressive, and sexually inappropriate (Chapter 4).

Coach vs. Parent, Judge, Critic, Taskmaster: A coach recognizes that although many players dream of being world champion few will achieve this. Nevertheless, the coach strives to bring the most out of each player. So too, a good mentor manages to encourage, motivate, challenge, redirect, and push without being an overcritical, micro-managing parent, a destructive critic, or a mindless taskmaster. A good coach, like a good mentor, develops your strengths and improves your weaknesses. A coach does this through high expectations, experience, character, strength, positive energy, confidence, feedback, insight, and enthusiasm. This does not mean that a coach never criticizes or is never a taskmaster – but it is positive and motivates the player to improve rather than feel useless. It also does not mean that a coach wears rose-colored spectacles and tells all the players they can be world champion. A coach gets players into great shape to compete, and then it is up to them to play to the best of their ability.

Confidante vs. Gossip: You expect your mentors to have the integrity to keep sensitive information private, but you also expect them to have the savvy to use sensitive information to solve a problem for you. This requires mutual trust.

Giver vs. Taker: A mentor gives and takes, but a good mentor gives rather than takes. Generous mentors give many things including time, ideas, advice, supplies, money, space, and stability. Selfish mentors give you just enough to do the job and use your labor to get their jobs done.

Mind-reader vs. Steamroller: Some mentors know what you are thinking – often before you know it. For example, they know when you are holding back because you are afraid to say something, when you have reservations about a plan, and when you are overwhelmed. Mentors with this social IQ use it to improve their coaching. Other mentors are unaware, or do not care what you are thinking. They are less flexible and focus exclusively on driving the project.

Plays well with others vs. Throws toys: Your scientific path will be easier if your mentor is mature and collaborative. Maturity does not automatically follow experience. Maturity includes reliability, evenness of temperament, ability to see the world from another's point of view, diplomacy, and not overreacting. It is difficult to work with a mentor who is up and down, sulks, gets upset about small things, demeans trainees, reprimands in public, or is passive-aggressive.

Able to let go vs. Hangs on: The source of much friction between mentors and mentees (and between parents and children) is transitioning to independence. Transitioning is hard for the mentor and the mentee. Traditionally, a complete parting of the ways was usual; after a fellowship you would take an idea, move to another institution, and develop an independent career. These days science is more collaborative and translational, and this "obligatory amputation" approach is seldom desirable. Moving is not just a question of packing your mice and hiring a new technician. A move early in your career can be dangerous (Chapter 4). You should maintain a support system through your mentor if you move.

A rush to independence can also be dangerous. A good mentor recognizes the mutual advantages of collaboration and helps you move to independence at the right speed. A bad mentor wants to take credit for every piece of your work and be last author on every paper you co-publish, forever.

Observes boundaries vs. Poor boundary recognition: There are boundaries to all relationships, but some mentors (and some mentees) have trouble recognizing them. The most common problems are about time (e.g., meetings at 7 p.m.), relationships (e.g., behaving like a friend rather a mentor), and requests (e.g., could you pick up my daughter from school?). If your mentor impinges on your boundaries, you should reset the boundary diplomatically (e.g., it is hard for me to meet at 7 p.m. because I have dinner with my family, would 7 a.m. suit you?). Remember, just as you have boundaries, so too does your mentor.

Can read a map vs. Wanders all over the place: Some mentors can think clearly and seem to predict the future. They understand your capabilities and choose projects and directions that have potential. Others scatter ideas everywhere, start and abandon projects, and choose dead-end projects.

Is responsible vs. Is not responsible for you: You are responsible for your success or failure. A good mentor understands this and helps you achieve your potential by providing excellent mentorship but not by taking responsibility for your success. A mentor could try to ensure your success by spoonfeeding you (e.g., writing your grants). This may sound attractive but it will only delay the point at which you fail or succeed, and it does not allow you to grow through struggle. If you subconsciously shift responsibility for your success to your mentor, you can develop an unhealthy dependency, a sense of entitlement, and unrealistic expectations. If you ever feel like blaming your mentor when things don't work out as you expected, remember that you are responsible for your career.

Clout: Your mentor's clout (influence, stature) provides intangible benefits and concrete advantages in resources, collaborations, and institutional support. Scientific clout provides benefits. Take an extreme example: if your mentor wins the Nobel prize, your career benefits tremendously by association. Political clout provides benefits. For example, if your mentor is the chair of department you benefit from that association. On the flip side, mentors with more clout often have more competing internal and external responsibilities and do not have as much time to mentor you. If you choose a mentor who also fills a senior leadership position, make sure the mentor has enough time for you. Some mentors with the most clout have large sink-or-swim labs where you are left to fend for yourself.

Signing on

Signing on with a mentor is not usually a formal signing but an agreement. By this stage, you will understand the mentor's expertise, style, reputation, and mentoring record. You will also know what your project is likely to be and the resources available. The mentor will understand your enthusiasm, commitment, availability, skills, and expectations. The intensity, duration, and expectations of the mentor-mentee relationship vary and evolve over time. For example, mentoring a medical student for a summer project is often a short-term commitment, but it could evolve into a long-term relationship. If your mentor is in "mentor-lite" mode, and you have different expectations, this can cause conflict. Some training programs have a formal written mentoring contract.

Mentoring contracts – written: Mentoring contracts usually specify concrete details and roles. For example, mentor will meet with mentee for one hour a week, provide 20 square feet of bench space, allow use of laboratory equipment, provide up to $200 of supplies and funding for travel to one meeting, assist with grant writing, and provide constructive feedback; mentee will start work at 8 a.m. on September 14, 2017, work hard, solicit feedback, maintain good communications, not divulge laboratory secrets, and so on.

I have mixed feelings about mentoring contracts. The major positive feature is that there can be no misunderstanding that the mentor is indeed a mentor. The major negative feature is that it is an artificial way of defining what should be a natural relationship. It is like having a marriage contract that specifies the responsibilities of each partner: Person A will take the trash out every Thursday; Person B will cook dinner every Monday. Also, people often regard mentoring contracts as just another piece of bureaucratic paper to sign rather than an opportunity to discuss expectations.

Mentoring contracts – unwritten: The agreement you reach with a mentor is more important than a written contract; this agreement is, in a sense, an unwritten contract. Rather than negotiating a written agreement stating who is going to take the trash out, it is more important to discuss each other's goals and expectations. It is also important to find out how the lab works, what the the unspoken "rules" of the lab are, and how you will develop independent projects that you can take with you when you leave. It is also a good time to set the stage for open discussion and feedback (Chapter 4): "It would be valuable if you give me feedback on how I am doing. It will help me improve and I won't view it as criticism."

Summary

1. Understand why you are doing research and what you want out of it.

2. Look for a mentor actively.

3. Look outside your comfort zone.

4. Research potential mentors before deciding.

5. If you plan a scientific career, your mentor must be experienced and successful, both as a scientist and as a mentor.

6. Your mentor must have enough time for you and invest in your career.

7. No mentor is perfect; choose a good fit.

8. Your mentor must be a top-notch scientist.

Resources

1. NIH RePORTER http://www.projectreporter.nih.gov/reporter.cfm

2. Tobin MJ. Mentoring: seven roles and some specifics. Am J Respir Crit Care Med 2004;170: 14-117 PMID:15242852.

3. Mirele-Cabodevila E. and Stoller JK. Research during fellowship – 10 commandments. Chest 2009;135:1395-1399 PMID:19420211.

4. Zerzan JT, Hess R, Schur E, Phillips RS, Rigotti N. Making the most of mentors; a guide for mentees. Academic Medicine 2009;84:140-144 PMID:19116494.

5. Bettmann M. Choosing a research project and a research mentor. Circulation 2009;119:1832-1835 PMID:19349336.

6. Huskins WC, Silet K, Weber-Main AM, Begg MD, Fowler VG Jr, Hamilton J, Fleming M. Identifying and aligning expectations in a mentoring relationship. Clin Transl Sci 2011;4:439-47 PMID:22212226.

Chapter 3

Choosing your project

Choose a mentor then a project

Potential mentors will ask about your scientific interests and tell you about theirs. Then, if there is common ground, a mentor might talk about possible projects. An important reason to choose a good mentor (Chapter 2) is that you are more likely to have a good project. A mentor might ask if you have ideas for a project. The question is to see if you are curious and can think; the mentor is usually not asking you to define the project you will do. Trainees are seldom responsible for thinking up a project, and a mentor is unlikely to let you loose on your own idea for two reasons. First, your project will spend the mentor's resources; therefore, it must derive from ideas that are already funded. Second, it takes years of experience to identify a good question and design an excellent project. Coming up with good questions is half the game; learning to turn good questions into testable hypotheses is the other half. A major goal of your training is to learn these skills.

What is the question and how will you address it?

When you discuss a research project, you should have a clear picture of the overarching idea, the question within that idea, and how the question will be answered by testing an hypothesis (Table). Vague projects ("We will measure a panel of biomarkers and I am sure we will see something for you to write up.") are high-risk.

Moving from ideas to hypotheses	
IDEA	Diet affects the outcomes of cancer.
QUESTION	Does diet affect the progression of breast cancer?
HYPOTHESIS	Test the hypothesis that in a prospective, randomized study a low fat (<10g/day) diet improves 5-year disease-free survival compared to a high fat diet (>50g/day) in 200 women with Stage 2 breast cancer.

What is a good question?

When you start research, you trust your mentor to come up with good questions. A measure of your growth and potential as an independent scientist is your ability to generate good questions. If you don't have a good question, why should anyone care about the answer? A good question and testable hypotheses are key for getting grants and publishing papers. A good question is NIFTI (**N**ew, **I**mportant, **F**easible, **T**estable, **I**nteresting) and has legs.

New

A new question identifies a knowledge gap. To recognize a knowledge gap you have to know the field and read widely. You cannot assume your mentor has researched the literature completely – that is your job. Your tasks are to define what is known, to identify interesting questions additional to the ones you propose to address, to evaluate the different methods people have used, to make sure your question is new and interesting, and to design your approach.

Important

If you are going to study something, why choose a trivial question? One way to assess the importance of a question is to ask yourself: *So what?* – the answer to that question should be compelling enough that a reviewer will think it important, no matter whether your study is positive or negative.

Feasible

Don't be overambitious; it always takes longer to do a study than you estimate. Consider the following questions. Do you have the right team? Are you using the right methods? Do you have the necessary time, patients, resources, and funding? Is the study really worth doing? Does the impact of the study justify the resources and effort you will expend?

Testable

Can you formulate your question into an hypothesis that is testable? An interesting question may not be testable given the resources you have.

Interesting

You will eventually have to "sell" a paper or a grant to reviewers, so choose an interesting question. Do not depend on your hypothesis having to be true to make the study interesting. A study is high-risk if you can only publish it if the answer comes out the way you hypothesize. A negative answer to a question should still be interesting and important. New questions on important topics are not automatically interesting; for example, the answer might provide minimal, incremental, and obvious information (the people-wear-more-clothes-in-cold-weather study).

Does the question have legs?

I thought I had come up with the concept of a project having legs, but recently I came across the same idea in an older paper (1). A project with legs teaches you important skills and techniques that advance your career and leads to further questions and studies. A project without legs is a one-off, dead-end study, or one that treats you as just a pair of hands.

Beware of the "quick and easy" project

If someone has a "quick and easy" project for you, run as fast as you can (mentors Alastair Wood and Wayne Ray). Few worthwhile projects are quick or easy. Weak projects often take just as much effort as strong ones. Even an apparently simple case-report takes a lot of time. Don't make quick or easy the reasons for choosing a project.

Beware of the "I am sure we can get an abstract out of it" project

Mentors sometimes feel pressure to have their trainees publish at least an abstract as evidence of research success. If a question is only good enough for an abstract (and not a paper), it is not worth doing. Abstracts rarely count for anything in an academic career. They serve some purpose on your CV if you have very few publications; however, abstracts that did not result in papers reflect poorly on someone who is more than a few years into a scientific career.

How many projects should you work on?

When I started research I was in Zimbabwe and my mentor there, Michael Gelfand, suggested that at any time I should be submitting a paper, writing another, working on another, and planning several. It was good advice. Research is a production line for discoveries, papers, and grants. If you have projects at different stages of development, you ensure long-term productivity and decrease the risk to your career if any particular project fails. Every mentor will tell you to focus, focus, focus. Indeed, focus on a project, focus on a research topic, and focus on your career are all critically important; however, even when you start research, you should have at least two active projects. When you are a mid-level investigator you will often have 6 or more active projects. You can think of your projects as an investment portfolio.

Your investment portfolio

There are several reasons not to put all your research eggs in one basket: some projects don't work out, some mature slowly, and some can only be done at certain times. Ideally, different projects will diversify your risk (high and low risk projects), flexibility (allow you to work when another project is inactive), science (teach you different but complementary skills – e.g., laboratory and clinical projects), date of maturity (some are published soon and others mature later), connections (collaborations outside your laboratory), and effort (you are not the main driver of every project).

Lack of focus vs. diversification

Almost certainly, the science you do in 10 years time will not be what you are doing now. Diversification is a rational branching from your existing research; it often involves new techniques or new diseases while maintaining your central focus. Diversification means that there is intellectual overlap between your projects. Thus, the reading you do for one project is part of the knowledge you need for another. It also means that data you generate for one project can be useful preliminary data to support a grant in a related area. In contrast to rational diversification, if you have a lot of different "interesting" projects unrelated to your central interest, it shows lack of focus. Appropriate diversification is good, but lack of focus is bad – your mentor can help you distinguish the two. The publications on your CV and biosketch (Chapter 21) will tell the story not only of your productivity but also of your focus and diversification.

How should your research relate to your clinical work?

If you are a clinician, it is ideal if your research is related to your clinical practice. This clinical niche provides you with a shared base of research and clinical literature and also makes it easier to recruit patients, obtain samples, interact with clinical colleagues, establish clinical expertise and a reputation in an area, and maintain your visibility as an expert at national meetings.

Good research projects do not materialize spontaneously

As you develop and transition to independence, you will choose your own projects. Each project you start is an investment – it costs you time, energy, and resources – all of which are finite. Therefore, the ability to think of good questions and to choose the best ones to develop into projects is a critical skill. Good questions grow from a combination of curiosity, creativity, extensive reading, and awareness. We all have many questions that at first seem interesting but later turn out to be pedestrian. I keep an ideas folder, and if I read an article that gives me an idea, I write the idea on the article and file it. Over months and years the folder grows, and from time to time I flip through it, read around some of the topics, and debate whether an idea is worth a study. Starting a project is easy but comes with long-term costs; as Mark Twain said, "It is easier to stay out than get out." Choose projects carefully.

Summary

1. When you start research, your mentor usually decides on the project; choose a proven mentor in the broad research area that you are passionate about.

2. Learning to ask good questions and turn them into testable hypotheses is a major goal of your training.

3. A good question is NIFTI (**N**ew, **I**mportant, **F**easible, **T**estable, **I**nteresting) and has legs.

4. Few projects are quick or easy.

5. Have a research portfolio that is focused but diversified.

6. Many questions are interesting, but few are worth pursuing.

Resources

1. Flockhart DA, Abernethy DR. Finding the right research question: quality science depends on quality careers. Clin Pharmacol Ther. 2008; 84(3):427-9. PMID: 18615005.

2. Mirele-Cabodevila E. and Stoller JK. Research during fellowship – 10 commandments. Chest 2009;135:1395-1399 PMID:19420211.

3. Zerzan JT, Hess R, Schur E, Phillips RS, Rigotti N. Making the most of mentors; a guide for mentees. Academic Medicine 2009;84:140-144 PMID:19116494.

4. Bettmann M. Choosing a research project and a research mentor. Circulation 2009;119:1832-1835 PMID:19349336.

Chapter 4
Interacting with your mentor

Interacting with your mentor – it's about the science

Your mentor will set the tone and expectations for interactions. You will interact in several settings; for example, doing the science (in the laboratory or clinic), planning and troubleshooting the science (lab meetings), and analyzing and presenting the science (preparing for talks, writing papers). Notice, interactions are about "the science." Your mentor is your scientific guide; initially at least, your interactions will center on the science – the common goal that binds you.

Improving your relationship with your mentor

All mentors and mentees have different strengths and weaknesses. Sometimes the relationship clicks, but as with any relationship, there will be irritations, unrealized expectations, and differences of opinion. Although your mentor is a major contributor, you should drive your side of the relationship. The more you contribute to the relationship (remember it's about the science), the more you will get out of it. Be proactive. Don't wait for your mentor to hand you something. Set goals for yourself, drive meetings by setting the agenda, solicit feedback, offer new ideas, ask questions, and get a scientific step ahead of your mentor. Ask for advice in specific areas. Learning to communicate is learning to see things from the other person's point of view. Solve problems before they become conflicts. You will learn these important skills from a good mentoring relationship.

Interacting with your mentor – ask for feedback

Your relationship with your mentor is based on communication. Some mentors (and some mentees) are better communicators than others. Communicating about your science is usually easy, communicating about your progress is more difficult, and asking for feedback is even more difficult. A mentor is reluctant to criticize you and may steer away from these conversations. One way to get feedback is to frame your question as a request for advice around goals or expectations. For example: "We had hoped to be half-way through the study but I am behind. Do you have any ideas how I can be more efficient?" Or, "One of my goals was to get a small grant, but my last two applications were triaged. Can you give me some pointers to improve my grant writing?" Some mentors will ask how they can more effective mentors. Rather than being negative: "You never do...," be positive: "It would be great if we could..." Although the word is "feedback," the process is easier and more helpful if everyone looks forward to find areas for future change and improvement rather than backward to past failures.

Mentee behavior that affects interactions with mentors

Good mentors value hard work, enthusiasm, taking ownership of a project, attention to detail, curiosity, following through, good relationships with others, and having realistic expectations. Bad mentors value mentees whose experiments "work" in that they come out as the mentor expected. If your relationship with your mentor is suboptimal, it can be helpful to look at your side of the equation – the side you can control. As Josh Fessel, one of the people who read a draft of the book, suggested, "Put yourself on the other side of the desk. Think about things from the standpoint of the mentor. How would you want your mentee to act? Are you doing that?" Self-reflection is good, but it can be difficult to be objective; others may see areas for improvement that are invisible to you. Solicit opinions from a trusted peer. Don't ask for judgment, ask for advice. "I want to do better. Can you tell me some concrete things I can do improve? I know it may be hard for you to tell me, but it would be a huge favor, so please be frank." If there are particular areas of your performance that worry you, ask about them directly. Remember, just as there is no perfect mentor, there is no perfect mentee. For all of us, insight is the first step to improvement, and enthusiasm, willingness to change, and hard work make up for our weaknesses.

Mentors have different styles

Mentors vary in how they interact – scientifically and socially. Some mentors point you in a scientific direction and then keep their distance; others keep a close eye on what you are doing. Similarly, some mentors are formal or even distant in their interactions, and others are sociable and casual. Your mentor's style is unlikely to change to accommodate you; find out what to expect before you start. Even so, you and your mentor will both need to adapt to have a successful relationship. Remember, no matter what the individual mentor's style, all good mentors have same drive – to do the best science possible. Don't mistake lightheartedness for lack of seriousness, or distance for lack of interest. Also, remember that your relationship and interactions with your mentor will evolve as you get to know each other and as your collaborative science advances.

Carve out some of your mentor's time but respect it

You must have a regular meeting on your mentor's calendar – once a week is usual. Make the most of this time. Prepare for the meeting and jot down an informal agenda – a list of things to discuss. This could include an experiment that is not working, a figure for a manuscript, who to ask about a new technique, and so on. If you don't have anything to discuss that week (from your point of view), email and see if your mentor still wants to meet. There is no point in meeting if there is nothing to discuss. If your lab meetings are small, they may fulfill many of the functions of one-on-one mentor meetings, and you may not need to meet as often.

Listening to your mentors

You will get advice from many different people besides your mentor. There is a skill to hearing an opinion, processing it, and finally acting. Advisors often understate opinions to avoid appearing dogmatic. After all, it is your grant, your paper, and your career – you must make the choices.

Listen to the subtext: Hearing the words is different from processing the message. For example, when a friendly internal reviewer reads a draft of your grant and says, "The Specific Aims could be tightened up," the reviewer is often really saying, "The Specific Aims are weak." There are several ways you could deal with a comment like this.

- You could ignore it because "tightening up" does not sound like a serious problem. If you do this, you will miss the opportunity to fix your grant.

- You could argue that the reviewer hasn't read the grant carefully. If you do this, the reviewer will seldom fight back. Volunteer reviewers do you a favor by reading your grant. They are seldom interested in defending their positions. Reviewers point out what they think the weaknesses are, and then the rest is up to you.

- You could ask the reviewer how to fix the problems. Reviewers get uncomfortable – they don't want to take responsibility for your Specific Aims or micromanage your application.

- You could ask the reviewer to explain what caught the critical eye. I think this is the best option because you are not asking the reviewer to identify a problem or to fix it – you are asking for insight into what caused a particular impression. Once you know that, you can identify the problem and fix it. If something grates on a reviewer, it should be a red flag for you.

Blind obedience is not listening: If you follow every piece of advice you receive, you will end up in a mess. It is difficult to recognize good criticism. For example, a mentor or a colleague can say something and you have an epiphany, an "aha moment," when you instantly recognize the problem, see the solution, and can, for example, improve your grant or paper immensely. More often, criticism sounds vague, conflicting, and difficult to evaluate. The more the criticism about papers or grants sounds like an unimpressed NIH study section (e.g., lacks logical progression, novelty is not clear, not mechanistic, not hypothesis driven, observational), the more carefully you should listen.

Mentor fatigue

Mentors get fatigued and stop repeating the same suggestions. If I make a suggestion a few times and nothing happens, I assume the person has heard, processed, and decided against the suggestion. If I am not the primary mentor, I stop making the suggestion; a trainee's ability to listen and act (or not) on advice is one factor that determines success. However, if I am the primary mentor, I will keep making what I think are crucial suggestions more and more forcefully.

Individual development plan

Despite all this discussion about how important mentors are, you are responsible for your career. You must direct your professional development, plan your career, and make sure you obtain the skills you need. Set concrete goals and milestones. Many NIH-funded training grants have an appropriate emphasis on an individual development plan (IDP) for each mentee (1). An IDP is an opportunity for you and your mentor to focus your thoughts on the big picture of your career trajectory. However, discussing an IDP should not be just an annual event; make it part of your regular routine with your mentor to asses where you are, where you want to be, and how to get there. Mentoring committee meetings (Chapter 5) will devote a lot of time to your development and this will also help focus your plans.

Have several mentors and keep them

You will need different mentors at different stages of your career, and you can have as many mentors as you need. You will generally have only one primary mentor at a time – this is the person who is most invested in overseeing your success. If you have developed a strong mentoring relationship with someone and move on to a new mentor, the relationship with the old mentor will endure, and you will find yourself seeking mentorship many years later. As you develop, you will surpass your previous mentors in some areas, and your student-teacher relationship will evolve into a relationship of equals. A colleague who is your equal or even your junior can be a wonderful mentor. The need for mentoring does not go away; the chief of your division has mentors that provide trusted guidance in difficult times.

Establishing independence from your mentor

Establishing independence and maintaining connections with mentors are both positive goals and should not be mutually exclusive. A good mentor recognizes your need for independence and will make sure that as you mature you direct some projects, publish some papers without the mentor, and are last author on some papers. The mentor will create some distance so that you have independent projects and papers that are clearly your work. This is often easier in the basic sciences. For example, in your fellowship you discover that the signaling pathways Jak-Stat and NF-kappaB are important in your area. You might pursue the Jak-Stat pathway and your mentor the NF-kappaB pathway. In this way you, "the Jak-Stat person," are clearly differentiated from your mentor. It can be more difficult to do this in clinical research because the number of logical next questions may be limited. For example, say you showed that salt sensitivity is an important regulator of cognitive function in the elderly (your mentor's idea originally). You can see how the logical next set of clinical studies is limited and it could be hard for you to differentiate from your mentor in this circumscribed area.

Splitting from your primary mentor

Losing a mentor or moving to a new mentor usually occurs for one of four reasons: 1) your mentor leaves; 2) you leave; 3) your science evolves towards a new primary mentor; or 4) your mentor is unsuitable.

1) Your mentor leaves

Academic scientists change institutions often, and it is not unusual for trainees to lose a mentor. As occurs with the unexpected ending of any important relationship, the first emotions are often despair, disbelief, and feelings of betrayal. If you have been invited to move with the mentor, the shock will be less sudden, and you will have had time to consider that decision. If you have not been invited, or if other components of your career make a move impossible, you might find out about the move only a few months before it happens. Whether you move with your mentor or stay behind, you will need to make several decisions quickly.

Should you go? If invited, moving with your mentor may seem the obvious choice, but you need to weigh the pros and cons from your point of view. The fact that your mentor is moving can lead to a useful but rude realization that your mentor does not revolve around you. This realization helps you to assess the move from your point of view. Aside from the inevitable delays that result from moving a laboratory, there are other things to consider. For example, what is your mentor's role at the new institution? A new dean may plan to keep a research operation going but be consumed by administration. Other relevant factors include equipment and other resources, collaborators, the new research environment and culture, your salary, moving a family, quality of life, and cost of living. A good mentor will put self-interest aside and help you decide what is best for you.

Should you stay? If you stay, you will need to find a new primary mentor. Sometimes the choice is obvious, and the approaching transition will appear easy. Nevertheless, it is important to meet with the outgoing and incoming mentors together so that there is a common understanding of expectations and responsibilities (e.g., who will fund and supervise incomplete studies). More often, choosing a new mentor seems like starting over. Although difficult to appreciate at the time, choosing a new mentor is an opportunity to diversify your research training and increase the pool of influential people invested in your career. The temptation is to choose the mentor best-qualified to help you complete your project. Rather, you should focus your choice on your future career not the immediate project, although they may be linked. Also, remember that when you apply for a career development grant you will need a K-quality mentor (Chapter 14).

2) You leave

Trainees leave institutions for various reasons. For example, lack of future opportunity at the home institution, to secure independence from the mentor, a "great package," and family reasons. Moving for a recruitment package that is attractive because of salary, lab space, or academic title is not a good idea (Chapter 23). These are ephemeral; your long-term future depends on building and securing your research career. As a developing academic researcher, you should move institutions only if it benefits your future long-term research career AND there is a great mentor for you at the new institution. A common scenario follows.

A postdoctoral fellow is highly successful, publishes several papers, and obtains a K-award. The fellow is keen to be independent and moves to another institution, attracted by a great recruitment package that includes promotion to assistant professor and independent research space. At the new institution it takes 18 months to get the research going and mentorship is weak. As a result, the new assistant professor is not productive and is not competitive for an R01 in year 4 of the K-award. The K-award and the recruitment package run out, and the institution asks the researcher to take on more clinical duties. This loss of protected time means less scientific productivity, and consequently often the downward spiral of an academic research career.

3) Your science evolves towards a new primary mentor

The most natural drive for you to move from one primary mentor to another is if the direction of your research changes. A good mentor will realize what is happening, encourage your progress, and remain involved but slowly transition mentoring responsibilities.

4) Your mentor is unsuitable

If you have problems with a mentor, you should try to fix or ameliorate them proactively. You can approach this through diplomatic discussion with the mentor and by changing the way you interact. If that does not work, or the problem is too serious or difficult for you to discuss with the mentor, seek confidential advice from a trusted peer and then from a senior faculty member responsible for career development. Most institutions have confidential counseling services, and many postdoctoral programs also have counselors. Take advantage of these. If none of this works, you face a major decision: stay or to leave. Don't make a decision to leave in a moment of temper. Weigh the pros and cons carefully and discuss the decision with an experienced advisor. If you transfer to another mentor or institution, it is best if you can leave on good terms with your mentor. If possible, avoid burning bridges or antagonizing people.

Chapter 2 discussed bad mentor behavior but did not include sexism and sexual harassment – two mentor behaviors that are devastating for mentees.

Sexism: Sexism occurs when people are treated differently because of their gender. Sexism is still a problem in academia; many studies show that women earn less than men for doing the same jobs and are less likely to be promoted or ascend to leadership positions (2). Most academic institutions recognize the problem and are trying to fix it. In contrast to institutional sexism, sexism in the mentor-mentee relationship is more difficult to quantify; however, it is just as pervasive. As with sexual harassment, sexism usually involves a male mentor and a female mentee. Some mentors, usually unconsciously, ascribe stereotypical characteristics to men (e.g., good at math, level-headed, independent, aggressive) and women (e.g., good verbally, excitable, needs support, caring). Such warped attitudes can affect every aspect of a mentee's development including the projects assigned, assessment of skills and achievements, and recommendations for advancement. In a study of K-awardees, 66% of women and 10% of men reported that they had personally experienced gender bias in professional advancement (3). Many women I know have suffered from this type of subtle discrimination, but unless there was something overt, many felt there was little they could do about the situation and tried to ignore it. Some tried to diplomatically correct stereotypic assumptions that affected specific components of their work. It is easier to identify and diplomatically confront overt sexism, for example, addressing women, but not men, as "honey," or complimenting women on their dress or physical appearance.

Sexual harassment: Sexual harassment in its most egregious forms includes sexual advances, using bribery, power, or threats to make sexual advances, and creating a hostile environment based on sexual innuendo or conversation.

Sexual harassment is common. Approximately 30% of female and 4% of male K-awardees reported they had personally experienced sexual harassment (3); women in this study experienced sexist remarks or behavior (92%), unwanted sexual advances (62%), subtle bribery (6%) or threats (1%) to engage in sexual behavior, and coercive advances (9%). If you face a situation like this, there are several possible responses, each with possible outcomes. The ideal outcomes are that the behavior stops, other mentees do not suffer the same behavior, your training and career continue successfully, and the mentor changes his ways. There are no data, but I suspect the types of outcomes in the scenarios below are more common than the ideal outcomes. An article by Kate Clancy in *Scientific American* describes her personal experience and the tremendous difficulties mentees face in this situation (4). Some responses to sexual harassment and their possible outcomes follow.

1) You confront: You could make it clear that his behavior is unacceptable and tell him to stop. He might or might not stop; either way, your working relationship could be altered to your detriment (e.g., resentment, poor reviews, unfounded criticism, micro-aggression, subtle character assassination).

2) You ignore it and try to live with it: You could pretend it never happened, or make light of it to avoid a scene that might damage your career. It is unlikely that the harassment will stop. Even if you later make it clear you find the attention unwelcome or the behavior offensive, the harassment could continue at the same level or even escalate.

3) You threaten: You could threaten to report him (or actually do so) to his superior. A threat might get him to stop, but he could take it out on you in ways that affect your career as in #1. A report would trigger an institutional investigation, and unless there is proof, there may be no resolution. Your working relationship will be destroyed.

4) You leave: You could decide there is no good outcome to the situation and seek a new mentor. Your current mentor could sabotage your efforts and future career.

Dealing with sexual harassment: As the scenarios illustrate, sexual harassment is one of the most difficult situations for a mentee to face and the outcome is often unsatisfactory. Each situation is different. Some behaviors are so egregious that they should be reported immediately; others may be borderline and resolve completely after you reset the boundaries. In all these situations I think two early actions on your part are important. First, politely but unequivocally reject the initial advance or behavior and set clear boundaries. Don't ignore it, it won't go away. For example, in response to an email saying how attractive you are and inviting you out on a date, decline categorically and say that your relationship is purely professional and that such overtures are unwelcome and unacceptable (5). Make sure you maintain rigid professional boundaries; don't engage in sexual banter to try and become accepted as part of the team, don't become the mentor's confidante, don't listen to his marital woes, and don't agree to meet outside of work to "discuss our situation." Second, act to protect yourself by 1) seeking advice and perspective, and 2) leaving a trail. Tell a confidential counselor what is happening and keep detailed, dated notes of events and conversations. Ideally, the person you tell should be bound by confidentiality, be part of your institution, and be independent of your mentor-mentee chain of command. Most institutions have Title IX counselors and employee health counselors available. Some people have had bad experiences with Title IX officials who acted to protect the institution and discredit the victim (6). The reason to speak to someone early is that if events escalate and you later decide to make a formal complaint there is a witnessed record of what the problem was and how you dealt with it. Without such a record, investigations can end up at at a "he said, she said" impasse unable to establish if anything untoward happened, and could even conclude that the victim overreacted or misinterpreted innocuous behavior. Perhaps the #MeToo movement will change culture, including academic culture.

Interacting with your mentor – romantic relationships

Some might think that a relationship between a mentor and a mentee is acceptable because both parties are adults. I view it like the relationship between doctors and patients. We expect professionalism, availability, expertise, insight, the ability to diagnose and prevent serious problems before they occur, deep caring, objectivity, setting aside of personal gain, advocating for the patient, and boundaries that preclude romantic and sexual involvement. We should have similar expectations of the mentor-mentee relationship. Mentors, like doctors, are in a position of power and should therefore not have romantic relationships with their mentees.

Many universities have policies forbidding such relationships between supervisors and subordinates and between faculty and their students. What if you believe the relationship will be important? You will either have to wait until you are working elsewhere, or you will have to choose between a mentor and a romantic relationship. If you choose the relationship, you will need to change mentors and restructure your career so that your ex-mentor does not supervise you and has no influence on your career. In this situation, a neutral senior person should oversee the dissolution of the mentor-mentee relationship and the hand-off of mentorship to a new mentor to ensure that there is no coercion or sexual harassment. This is not straightforward and will often involve division and department heads.

Summary

1. Interactions with mentors center on science.

2. Every work meeting should have an agenda (not necessarily a written agenda).

3. Learn to listen to the subtext and read between the lines.

4. All mentors and mentees have quirks.

5. Learning to work together is a process that often involves change.

6. Keep your relationship with your mentor after you develop independence.

7. You will have several mentors and can have as many as you need.

Resources

1. FASEB site "MyIDP" http://myidp.sciencecareers.org/.

2. Jena AB, Khullar D, Ho O, Olenski AR, Blumenthal DM. Sex differences in academic rank in US medical schools in 2014. JAMA 2015;314(11):1149-58. PMID:26372584;

3. Jagsi R, Griffith KA, Jones R, Perumalswami CR, Ubel P, Stewart A. Sexual harassment and discrimination experiences of academic medical faculty. JAMA. 2016;315(19):2120-1. PMID:27187307.

4. From the Field: Hazed Tells Her Story of Harassment. Kate Clancy, 2012 https://blogs.scientificamerican.com/context-and-variation/from-the-field-hazed-tells-her-story-of-harassment/

5. Jahren, Hope. She wanted to do her research he wanted to talk feelings. Opinion Piece. New York Times March 14, 2016.

6. A blog describing bad experiences with Title IX investigations. https://tenureshewrote.wordpress.com/2015/09/21/title-ix-a-step-by-step-guide/

7. Zerzan JT, Hess R, Schur E, Phillips RS, Rigotti N. Making the most of mentors; a guide for mentees. Academic Medicine 2009;84:140-144 PMID:19116494.

8. Detsky AS, Baerlocher MO. Academic mentoring--how to give it and how to get it. JAMA. 2007;297:2134-6 PMID:175073

Chapter 5

Your mentoring committee

Why have a mentoring committee?

Mentees dread mentoring committees. They avoid calling meetings and treat them as ritual public disembowelment. This is a mistake. Your mentoring committee is not "big brother" or a panel of judges; it is a group of people committed to helping you succeed. The committee is on your side, and its members have all faced the same challenges you face. If you are serious about a career in research, you must have a mentoring committee. Here are some reasons.

- The committee sees the picture of your career trajectory while you are more focused on the day-to-day battles.

- The whole is greater than the sum of its parts (Aristotle). Meeting individually with members is not the same as having a committee meeting. When a group of smart people sit in the same room and focus on the same question there is synergy.

- The committee expands your mentor's clout and your circle of influence.

- The committee can help with mentoring issues, for example, by diplomatically suggesting to your mentor that it is time for you to be last author on some papers.

- The committee carries more weight than your mentor. For example, if your division chief is pressuring you to do too much clinical work, your committee can intervene.

- The committee can help you in any way you need (e.g., discuss Specific Aims for a grant, review your grant, introduce you to someone, solicit speaking invitations, advise about career choices).

Who should be on your mentoring committee?

A mentoring committee often has 3 or 4 members with deep expertise in your scientific and career areas. If it has too many members, it will be hard to get them together and there will not be enough time for them to say what they think. The path of least resistance is to choose some senior collaborators. They may not be the best people to guide you. Also, trainees sometimes choose inexperienced faculty – because "they are more in touch with where I am in my career." There are some advantages; less experienced people do help keep the more senior members grounded, but I think mentoring committees work best if all the members have weight and are outstanding scientists. You can invite junior colleagues to lunch and discuss career questions. Choose mentors for specific reasons (e.g., great expertise in genetic research). It is helpful if the people you invite know you or your mentor, and there is no point choosing someone who does not show up and is not committed to helping you. Discuss the membership of the committee with your mentor. If you are in a clinical division, it is often a good idea to have the chief of the division on your committee. Even if the chief is not a scientist, he or she can influence your future scientific career significantly.

Your mentor and the mentoring committee

Your mentor will almost always attend meetings but is often not a member of the committee. With this structure the committee can be independent and advise both you and your mentor. It is useful if the committee has a defined chairperson who steers the discussion.

What do I do for a mentoring committee meeting?

Schedule the meeting: You call the meetings and direct them. Meetings usually occur at 6-12 month intervals; schedule them a long time ahead – it can be difficult to find a time when all members are available. Two documents are useful to help guide the meeting: a progress report and an agenda.

Circulate a progress report before the meeting: The committee wants to know your academic rank, current and pending funding, how you are spending your time, what you are working on, how productive you are, your achievements, plans, timeline, and where you need help. Your progress report should be bulleted or in point form and 1-2 pages long with clear headings. An example follows.

> <u>**Mentoring Committee Meeting**</u>
> **Mary Smith M.D, MSCI. 9/1/2017 at 3 pm room 123 Building A.**
>
> **Rank:** Instructor (appointed 7/1/2013) Div of Pulmonary Medicine, physician-scientist track
>
> **Mentor:** George Green PhD
>
> **Time Allocation:**
> *Research* 85% *Clinical* 18% (weekly outpatient clinic Wednesday 2-5 pm; attending consult service 4 weeks/year) *Teaching* 0% *Administrative* 2% (1 hour meetings for resident research committee every 2 weeks)
>
> **Current Funding:**
> PI Smith, Mary (60% effort)
> American Thoracic Society career development award (7/1/15 – 7/1/17) $75,000
> Role of interleukin-1 in clinical progression of pulmonary hypertension
> PI Green, George (20% effort)
> RO1 HL12345 (1/3/2014- 2/28/2019)
> Inflammation in pulmonary hypertension

Current Research:

- mostly working on Aim 1 of my ATS award – established the animal model and completing quantification of IL-1 expression in pulmonary vasculature.
- helping with a clinical proof-of concept study of mycophenolate as a treatment for pulmonary hypertension
- minor helping hand in a fellow's project. She is using my animal model to study the pulmonary microvasculature response to a PDE4 antagonist.

Honors: My abstract "IL1 expression in the human lung" was awarded an ATS travel scholarship for the 2017 national meeting.

Publications in last year:

Smith M, Brown B, Green G. Pulmonary microvascular remodeling after inhibition of interleukin 28. *Pulm Circ Physiol* 2016;34:240-5.

Smith M, Black B, Green G. Enhancement and maintenance of pulmonary microvasculature remodeling by inhibition of inflammation associated calcium signaling. *Thoracic Res* 2017 (in press).

Indigo I, **Smith M**, Black B, Green G. Pulmonary microvasculature flow-mediated dilation is impaired by inflammation. *Proc Nat Acad Lung Science* (Revision submitted).

Smith M, Brown B, Green G. Adipokines affect pulmonary microvascular remodeling (preparing, should be ready to submit in 2 months).

Funding Goals: Submit K application March 2018; submit same application as a VA Career Development Award.

Other Goals next 12 months: Get the adipokine paper published. Complete Aim 1 of the ATS grant in the next few months and submit an abstract to the American Heart meeting (due March), have paper submitted by July.

Specific questions for Committee: I would like to spend most of this meeting getting your feedback about the draft Specific Aims (attached) for my K-award application.

Circulate an agenda before the meeting: The agenda is brief but helps to structure the meeting. For example, let's say you want to spend most of the time discussing the Specific Aims for your K application. If you don't have an agenda and you start the meeting with the latest results of your experiments, the committee could spend the whole hour discussing the nuances of your fascinating experiments. An example agenda follows.

Agenda Mentoring Committee Meeting

Mary Smith M.D, MSCI. 9/1/2017 3-4 pm room 123 Building A.

1. I will present highlights of progress (Progress document attached) (5 minutes)

2. I will show new data that will support K application (5 minutes) and present the rationale and potential Specific Aims (draft attached) for K-award (10 minutes)

3. Committee discusses Specific Aims

4. Committee chair summarizes

Arrive early and come prepared: Don't be late for the meeting. Arrive a few minutes early and if you have slides have them up. Have spare copies of the agenda, your progress report, and any material you specifically want to discuss (e.g., draft Aims). Take a copy of your CV in case anyone wants to look at it.

Help drive the meeting: This is your meeting to direct as you wish. If people get sidetracked you can politely revert to the agenda. For example, "That is really helpful. Thank you. I wanted to make sure we had enough time to discuss my draft Specific Aims so it would be great if we can leave time for that." Take notes during the meeting.

Close the meeting: Some mentoring committees will ask you (and sometimes your mentor) to leave the room for a few minutes so that they can have a private discussion. If that happens, after you return the chair will usually close the meeting by summarizing the committee's main thoughts. If the chair does not close the meeting with a summary, you can close the meeting by summarizing what you think the main points were and thanking everyone for their time and expertise.

Write a report: It is helpful for you to keep a brief written summary of what the committee discussed.

Summary

1. If you are serious about an academic career, have a mentoring committee.
2. It is your responsibility to call the meetings.
3. The point of the meetings is not to criticize but to guide and coach you.
4. Circulate your progress report and an agenda before the meeting.
5. Direct the meeting to areas where you want guidance.

Resources

1. Guise JM, Geller S, Regensteiner JG, Raymond N, Nagel J. Building interdisciplinary research careers in women's health program leadership. Team mentoring for interdisciplinary team science: lessons from K12 scholars and directors. Acad Med. 2017;92(2):214-221. PMID: 27556675.

Chapter 6

Time management

TIME IS ONE OF YOUR MOST VALUABLE ASSETS. It is finite and you must manage it actively. You will always be too busy; there are never enough hours in the day, and there is always too much to do. You can either "wing it" with an intuitive allocation of time (as most people do), or manage your time actively so that you are most productive in the areas that matter.

Where does your time go?

To manage your time you first need to know where it goes. Keep track of how you spend your time over a week. You needn't log every minute obsessively, but you do need specific details, not back-of-the-envelope estimates. You are looking for both big commitments that use chunks of time and smaller tasks that use more time than you thought. You are also looking for wasted time; 30 minutes of a 10-hour day is 5% of the day. There will be some surprises and you will almost certainly find that you are spending less time doing research than you thought. Once you know how you are spending your time, you can make a plan.

Planning how to spend your work time – the big picture

Consider the demands on your work time and divide them into three or four broad categories. For example, these might include research, clinical duties, teaching, and administrative duties. Then allocate the proportion of your time that should be spent on each activity. The proportions you allocate indicate the direction of your career, because how you spend your time determines your career track (Chapter 1). If you are on a research track, allocate your time as follows.

First, allocate at least 80% of your time to research: To be successful in research you need to spend most of your time doing research. One major goal of time management is to ensure that you spend enough time doing research. This is particularly true in the early phases of your career when you are learning techniques, establishing yourself as an investigator, and building a reputation. Many career development awards require you to spend 80% of your time doing research. This is appropriate. Don't try to cut corners in creative ways. For example, some people fool themselves that based on a 40 hour week, 32 hours of research fulfills the 80% research goal. If you actually work a 60 hour week and use 32 hours for research then 28 hours (almost 50% of what you are doing) is spent on clinical and other activities. If your goal is to be a physician-scientist or a tenure-track scientist, you are more likely to succeed if you spend at least 80% of your time doing research.

Then, divide the remaining 20% of your time between the other commitments: The rest of your activities can occupy no more than 20% of your time. Pencil these activities into your calendar first, because they tend to be fixed and predictable (e.g., a weekly clinic or meeting). Be honest with yourself – a morning clinic running from 8 a.m. to 1 p.m. is seldom a 5-hour commitment. There are letters to dictate, calls to make, administrative meetings, and so on. If your non-research commitments occupy more than 20% of your time, you should reconsider either your time allocation or your goal to be an independently-funded scientist.

Make sure everyone is working from the same big picture: Make sure that your big picture is compatible with the picture your colleagues and superiors have. For example, if you plan to spend 15% of your time on clinical activities, your division chief needs to support that plan. It is far easier to reach an agreement when you start a job than it is to renegotiate later. Also, if you agreed on a plan initially, it is easy and appropriate for you to return later and ask for relief from any added clinical, administrative, or teaching loads. However, the guaranteed protected time you were offered when you were appointed as a new faculty member will expire unless you obtain research grants to support your research career.

Planning how to spend your work time

The small details: Once you have set your big picture time allocation, you can focus on day-to-day time management. You should plan each day to get the most out of it. To plan the day you need to know what tasks you need to do, how long they will take, and their individual time-lines. This means you must plan across years, months, weeks, and days for different intertwined tasks. The easiest approach is to break tasks into achievable units and plan those. For example, if it is February and you are planning to submit a new grant early next year, the outline of tasks and their time-line could look like this.

10. Submit grant (January next year).

9. Have grant reviewed internally and make changes (November).

8. Have grant written (October).

7. Get preliminary data on at least two patients for grant (August).

6. Get the key data supporting the idea for the grant written up and submitted (June).

5. Get Specific Aims reviewed by mentor and committee and redraft (May).

4. Draft Specific Aims for grant and read literature around them (April).

3. Get IRB approved for studies to generate preliminary data for the grant (March).

2. Do two more experiments for #6 (next week).

1. Order new reagents and make buffers and label tubes for #2 (tomorrow).

Have long term plans: To sustain your academic career, you must maintain continuous funding. This takes careful planning. Grant applications have two predictable characteristics that you must plan for: 1) most applications are not funded, and 2) there is a big time gap between when you submit the application and eventual funding. You can submit most categories of NIH grants three times a year. Take the example of an RO1 you submit in February: it will usually be reviewed in June-July, and proceed to Council in August-October with an earliest start date of December. You can see that even for the unusual grant that sails straight through there is almost a year from submission to receiving the money. Considering that few grants are funded on the first application and that NIH often delays the start date, you should have plans and goals that stretch 1, 2, and 5 years ahead.

Make lists: Plan each day using lists. Some people have an excellent intuitive clock and calendar, others make lists, and others lurch from deadline to deadline. Lists help me keep track; also, I find it very satisfying to cross a task off my list when I have finished it. Take 5 minutes in the morning to plan your day and apportion 30-minute blocks of time to tasks according to their priority. There will be some tasks that you have to accomplish today, (e.g., meet the deadline to submit a letter-of-intent) and others with a more distant time horizon. The trick is to juggle both the urgent (and often more mundane tasks) and those that are more distant and often less well-defined. When you are working hard and struggling to complete day-to-day tasks, it is important not to lose sight of tasks that support your distant goals. Set yourself deadlines for important tasks and meet them.

The urgent/important matrix: Stephen Covey described a four quadrant urgent/important matrix to classify demands on time (1) that some people find useful.

Quadrant 1 is *urgent and important*; for example, your patient has chest pain, your grant deadline is tomorrow, your tax returns are due today. You have to take care of these immediately. If too many of these emergencies are self-inflicted, you can lessen the daily chaos with better planning (why didn't you do your tax returns earlier?).

Quadrant 2 is *not urgent but important*; for example, reading journal articles, thinking about a grant, learning a new technique, building relation-ships, exercising. Your goal is to spend more time on quadrant 2 tasks.

Quadrant 3 is *urgent but not important*; for example, many of the emails and texts we receive, someone coming into your office to ask you something trivial, and some meetings. You can alter your behavior and that of others to minimize this quadrant.

Quadrant 4 is *not urgent and not important*; for example, surfing the internet, gossiping. Spend little time in quadrant 4.

Focus intensely on one task for a block of time

It is difficult to focus intensely for more than 20-30 minutes, and it is impossible to focus intensely on more than one task. Multitasking is inefficient, so if you have three 20-minute blocks allocated to working on a paper, don't answer the phone, don't let people into your office, don't make calls or look at text messages, and don't check the latest news on the internet. You can fit all of these other activities into your working day, but not into a working block that is allocated to something else. You will find it more efficient to allocate a separate block of time, or to use a break between blocks, to answer your email and make calls. At the end of a block of time, take a short break and do some of the things that would have distracted you. Then start a new block. This is the way many people study for exams – working intensely for a block of time and then taking a break. Carrying this approach into the work day will make you more efficient. If you keep a calendar that shows how you used your blocks of time, you can look back and see how you are actually spending your time and make adjustments if necessary.

Don't waste time

There are many different ways to waste time without realizing it. One way to identify time-sinks is to ask the following questions.

- *Why am I doing this task?* Every task should be compatible with your mission in some way – it should advance your career through research, clinical work, leadership, or good citizenship.

- *Am I the right person to do this task?* Delegating some tasks will save you a lot of time, but delegating the wrong task to the wrong person can cost you time. When you start research you may have little support and not be able to delegate – you make buffers, culture cells, inject mice, review medical records, fill out IRB forms, recruit and screen patients, and make appointments.

- *Is this the right amount of time for this task?* Are you spending too long on a task that does not require perfection?

- *Am I doing the task efficiently?* If you are not focused exclusively on the task, you are not efficient. Deal with something once, rather than starting it and then procrastinating so that you have to return to it and waste time reorienting yourself. It is more efficient to complete a task when the information is fresh in your mind. It is more efficient to write papers or grants in intense blocks of time over days or weeks than in scattered hours over months. Meetings should have an agenda, although it need not be written (I once heard someone say, "No agenda, no attenda!"). Meetings should be short and focus on the point of the meeting; few need to be longer than 30 minutes, and almost none longer than 60 minutes.

- *Am I wasting time unrelated to the task?* Don't waste time doing things unrelated to your tasks (e.g., chatting, gossiping, surfing the internet, and so on).

Waste some time

You should not plow through your tasks like an automaton. Deviating from your schedule can be very productive. I have developed many new insights and collaborations from an unexpected chat with a colleague. Creativity and new ideas often come from unexpected places – it helps if your mind and time are open to the unexpected, and if you are aware of situations where good things are more likely to happen. If someone you respect wants to see you with a burning idea, but you can't find a slot your calendar for 3 weeks, that idea will disappear.

Be considerate of your time and other people's time

A closed door respects your time: If you are working intensely for a block of time you should be considerate to yourself and protect that time. Close the door. Put up a "Do Not Disturb" sign if you have to. An "open door policy" sounds attractive, but there are few benefits to allowing people to wander in and out of your office when you want to work. There are very few situations where someone needs to see you immediately. It is better to give people time on your calendar when it suits you and know why they are coming to see you (the agenda). If you are uncomfortable denying people rapid access, put a sign on your closed door that directs people to your next break; for example, "If you need to see me today I will be free for 5 minutes at 10.30."

Punctuality respects other people's time: Punctuality is important. You respect other people's time when you arrive on time. This is particularly important if you work with collaborators who are punctual, and if a meeting cannot start until everyone is present – in that case, everyone is hostage to the tardy.

How many hours do I need to work?

Trainees often ask how many hours a week a researcher needs to work. It is important to put the hours in, but it is more important to work efficiently and effectively. There is no magic number of hours that ensures success, and there are frightening, probably apocryphal, anecdotes about famous scientists who sleep 3 hours a night (they are often asleep in seminars). Nevertheless, successful researchers do tend to work more than less successful ones; a research career is not an easy option and will not thrive on a 9-5 approach. Almost every successful researcher takes work home sometimes or works on the weekends (as do most successful clinicians). A survey of K-awardees found that men and women said they worked an average of 59 and 54 hours a week, respectively; 59% of men and 35% of women worked more than 60 hours a week (2). Of K-awardees who had children, women spent 8.5 hours a week more than men on domestic activities (2).

Time is finite but flexible

One of the biggest benefits of a research career is flexibility. A researcher can schedule time off during the working week much more easily than someone with clinics booked months ahead. For example, if you plan ahead, you can go to your child's birthday party and then do some extra work at home that evening.

Balancing life

In any demanding career it is difficult to balance life so that work and home both run harmoniously. You will need to develop a personal approach to the problem. Your family responsibilities and the things that are important to you guide your decisions. Just as you define priorities to manage your work time, you should define the priorities for your social time and then use your time management skills to organize them. If you have a family, it will be important to discuss your approach so that everyone aligns priorities, divides tasks, and makes big career decisions together. These details will vary for each family, but what is important is that you make time for your social and family commitments. You and your family will have to find the right balance that works for everyone.

You cannot work at full speed all the time

There are times when you have to work at full speed, but you can't sprint all the time. For example, if you have a grant deadline, you might have to work late into the night. But, if you do this all the time, you will burn out. An academic career needs time for reading widely and thinking reflectively – that is how you get inspiration and ideas. Be aware of how fast you are running and set an appropriate pace. Make time for relaxation; paradoxically, it might improve your work. I have a tendency to expand my work to fill the time available (Parkinson's Law), so having less time available often makes me more efficient. Also, science is about being creative, and you cannot be creative if you are burnt out. Relaxation, in addition to recharging your batteries, can spur creativity. Some of my best ideas arrive out of nowhere when I am jogging or walking the dog.

Learn to say NO

At the beginning of your career it feels like a great honor when someone asks you to write a review article, give a talk, teach a course, see a patient, or review a paper. Some of these tasks may be congruent with your career goals, but you should not get swamped and derailed from your main purpose. For example, review articles increase your visibility in an area, but they count for little on the physician-scientist track. If you write too many review articles it diverts you from publishing original scientific papers. Balance is important. In the early years of your research career, avoid administrative, teaching, or committee responsibilities. Keep track of your time allocation with an eye on your core focus and long-term goals and learn to decline invitations diplomatically.

Saying No directly (diplomatically): It can be difficult to say no to your boss. Let's say your division chief asks you to give some lectures to the medical students, or to do someone's clinic for 3 months, or to be a liaison person with the outpatient administrative team. The simplest way to decline is directly, unambiguously, briefly, and politely, "Thanks for asking me but I am sorry my schedule is really full right now and I cannot take that on."

Saying No indirectly (diplomatically): It can be difficult to say no directly. A diplomatic option is to decline with a vague and negative qualifier. For example, "Thanks for asking me, but my plate is really full right now and I don't think I will be able to do it, but I could get back to you if you like." Then, unless the person comes up with a strong request for you to get back in touch, you are off the hook. Usually the person will say something like, "Let me ask around and I will get back to you if need be." Again, you are free. Remember, requests are often hierarchical; the person asking you was asked by someone else and usually just wants to move the task onto anyone else's plate. The person asking you has little personal interest in who does the job, and if you decline, will usually move on to someone else and not get back to you. If the person does get back to you, then it is time to decline directly. If someone makes requests that are incompatible with your goals and won't take no for an answer, you should speak to your mentor about the problem. Remember, if an email request to perform a task is copied to several people, the simplest way to decline is simply not to reply. Of course, if the email is sent to just you or a couple of people, you should reply.

Learn to say YES

Despite what I have just said, and even if your plate is full, there are times when you must say yes, because it is the right thing to do for your career, or because it is your responsibility as a good academic citizen (Chapter 26). For example, you are invited to co-author a review article for an extremely high-impact journal; you have been funded by the local chapter of the Heart Foundation and they invite you to attend a workshop for patients; a Nobel prize-winner asks you to co-author a book chapter. Also, until you have been promoted (Chapter 20), it is a good idea to say yes to invitations to give talks at outside institutions and to sit on an NIH study section.

Is the juice worth the squeeze?

One way to save time is to avoid tasks that are not worth doing or that consume too much time relative to their yield. Ask yourself if the juice is worth the squeeze (mentor Wayne Ray). Every activity we undertake consumes time and effort (squeeze) and yields something (juice). I approach participation in activities (studies, papers, collaborations, committees) by asking myself (often subconsciously) several questions: Why should I do this? Why should I not do this? What are the best, worst, and likely outcomes? These questions help me decide how important a task is and how to spend my time most effectively.

Common reasons researchers get into a mess with time management

- Not spending enough time doing research.
- Unwittingly drifting to non-research activities (e.g., too much clinical time). People vote with their feet: too much clinical time may be your feet voting for a change in career goals.
- Losing sight of long-term goals and their timeline.
- Procrastination.
- Overload (both self-inflicted and from superiors).
- Not prioritizing.
- Frittering time away on unimportant activities.
- Not allowing for a predictable time lag (e.g., the lag between applying for funding and receiving it).
- Not setting time-lines, goals, and deadlines for tasks.

Summary

1. Know where your time goes.

2. Allocate your time according to your priorities.

3. Manage your time actively.

4. Plan ahead and set deadlines.

5. If you want a career as an academic researcher, spend more than 80% of your time doing academic research.

6. Don't waste your time.

7. Don't waste other people's time.

8. Pace yourself.

Resources

1. Stephen R. Covey. The 7 habits of highly effective people. Simon & Schuster; Anniversary edition, 2013.

2. Jolly S, Griffith KA, de Castro R, Stewart A, Ubel P, Jagsi R. Gender differences in time spent on parenting and domestic responsibilities by high-achieving young physician-researchers. Ann Intern Med 2014;160:344-53.

Chapter 7
Writing a paper – what goes where

Writing is important – published papers and successful grant applications are measures of success and productivity. You will notice that the approaches to writing a good paper and a good grant (Chapter 12) are very similar and hinge on a new, important question and a clear, logical exposition.

Traditionally, scientific writers learn to write by mimicking papers they admire. The lack of formal teaching is a problem because publishing research papers is an arcane game. The reviewers of your papers will know the rules. It is important that you too learn the rules so that you don't mark yourself as incompetent.

The components of a paper

Papers have a standard format: 1) Title page, 2) Abstract, 3) Introduction, 4) Methods, 5) Results, 6) Discussion, 7) Acknowledgements/Conflict of Interest/ Funding sources, 8) References, 9) Tables and Figures, and 10) Figure legends. If you refer to the "Instructions to Authors" section on the website of your target journal, you will find additional details specific to that particular journal. Most journals require that submissions be double-spaced with a least 1 inch margins and sequentially numbered pages. When you submit online you often have to upload the body of the manuscript and the Tables and Figures separately. The journal then reconstructs the full paper and sends it to reviewers in a pdf format. I will describe the components of a paper in the order in which they appear, but this is usually not the order in which you write them.

1) The title page

An example of a title page follows. Don't worry if all the components of the title page don't fit on one page. You can extend onto the second page, but make sure the next section – usually the abstract – starts on its own page. Here is an example of a title page.

Variation in the beta-adrenoceptor gene alters the effect of atenolol on plasma insulin and glucose

George Grey, MD; Michael Maroon, Ed E. Emerald, MD

Short title: Genetics and atenolol effect on insulin and glucose

From the Departments of Medicine and Pharmacology, Division of Clinical Pharmacology (G.G., E.E.E.), Greenish University School of Medicine, New York, NY; Department of Pharmacology, University of Ceil, London, England (M.M.)

Pages and Word Count: 29 pages including 2 Figures and 2 Tables, 3144 words

Correspondence to: Ed Emerald, MD, Division of Clinical Pharmacology, 542 Building 2, Greenish University School of Medicine, New York, NY 10000. Phone +1-321-987-6543, Fax: +1-321-987-2234. Email ed.e.emerald@greenish.edu

The title page – choosing a title: The title of your paper is the first thing an editor, reviewer, or casual reader sees, so give it thought. Your title should communicate your whole paper succinctly. From the title alone an informed reader (such as an editor or reviewer) is already judging novelty, importance, and suitability for the journal. There are 3 basic approaches to titles: 1) *Describe the battle* (The effect of drug X on Y); 2) *Declare victory* (Drug X increases Y); and 3) *Declare you won the war* (Drug X markedly increases Y and cures cancer). Some authors prefer to telegraph their positive results (Approach 2), and this does produce a more catchy title. However, some journals (e.g., the *New England Journal of Medicine)* require that the title describe what you did, rather than what you found (Approach 1). Approach 3, the equivalent of shouting from the rooftops, is seldom appropriate and will antagonize reviewers.

The title page – authors: The list of authors contributes only a few lines to a 30 page manuscript but can get you into a terrible mess. Disagreements about authorship can lead to bitter, long-lasting academic feuds. You can make enemies by omitting people who believe they should have been authors and by the order in which you place the authors.

Who should be an author – the criteria: According to the widely used International Committee of Medical Journal Editors (ICMJE) recommendations quoted below, an author must meet all four of the following requirements (1):

1. *Substantial contributions to the conception or design of the work; or the acquisition, analysis, or interpretation of data for the work; AND*
2. *Drafting the work or revising it critically for important intellectual content; AND*
3. *Final approval of the version to be published; AND*
4. *Agreement to be accountable for all aspects of the work in ensuring that questions related to the accuracy or integrity of any part of the work are appropriately investigated and resolved.*

Everyone who meets these 4 requirements, and no one who does not, should be an author. Generally, it is obvious who the authors of a paper should be, but sometimes deciding what constitutes a "substantial contribution" can be difficult.

Who should be an author – application of the ICMJE criteria: Should a technician who did the assays be an author? What about research nurses? And the research fellow who started the study three years ago but left before any patients were enrolled? My approach to these three scenarios (all real) is as follows. Technicians are potential authors if they contribute substantial intellectual content (e.g., developed or modified an assay, or used a non-standard assay they optimized). The technician who measured serum potassium would not be considered for authorship, but the one who developed a new antibody assay would. Research nurses are also potential authors if they contribute substantial intellectual content (e.g., developed new questionnaires or better ways of doing the study). A research nurse who simply follows a protocol and recruits patients would not be a potential author. The research fellow who started the project three years ago would be a potential author if he or she had contributed intellectually, even if no patients had been recruited, because refining the hypothesis and writing the IRB application and protocol are a substantial intellectual contribution, even if this was before the first patient enrolled.

Who should not be an author? Your boss should not be an author merely for being your boss. A medical student who visited the lab a few times does not qualify for authorship even though "giving him a paper would be great for his CV." If you follow the four ICMJE requirements for authorship, things are usually clear. As a trainee, if I was uncertain whether someone qualified for authorship, I asked the senior author and co-authors, and if I was still unclear, I asked the senior author to check with the person directly. That email can be something like this: "We are finally writing up…. I have lost track of the contributions everyone made to pieces of the study and I wanted to check if, based on your contributions, you should be an author." I like this approach because it is direct and it makes clear that the person asked must qualify for authorship and assume the accompanying responsibilities.

Ghost-authorship is unethical: Ghost-authors are people who meet the criteria for authorship but are missing from the list of authors. This practice is most often associated with review articles from the pharmaceutical industry; the review was conceived and written by a professional writing company (paid by the pharmaceutical company), but figurehead authors (often academic researchers) take credit for this unacknowledged work. If you are approached by someone to write a review article, make sure that you write the article independently and that your accompanying conflict of interest (Chapter 27) statement is accurate.

Professional writers must be visible: There is nothing wrong with a professional writing company helping with a manuscript, particularly for authors who have difficulties with English. However, the acknowledgments section of the paper must specify the exact role of the professional writers and who paid them. Remember, the authors, not the writing company, are responsible for the paper. Review articles are particularly open to bias because they contain nuanced opinion. Avoid writing a review article commissioned by a pharmaceutical company or co-authoring one drafted by a writing company, even if those facts are declared. The worst abuses have occurred when a writing company has ghostwritten a paper and an academic scientist has paraded as the author.

Do not gift authorship: Gift authorship is when someone who does not qualify for authorship is "given" authorship. Authors do this out of respect, friendship, the hope that if they include people on a few of their papers they will do likewise, not wanting to give offence, and many other reasons. Don't do it.

All authors must sign: All your co-authors will have contributed to writing the paper, but they should also all approve the final version. Most journals, at some stage in the publication process, ask all authors to sign a statement accepting the responsibilities of authorship and to declare their conflicts of interest. Never forge anyone's signature no matter how reasonable it seems. If Dr. Grey is climbing Mt. Everest and is out of contact, you should explain that to the editor rather than sign for Dr. Grey, even though you are sure she would have wanted you to sign.

Who should be first author? The first author is usually the person who did the most work and wrote the first draft. Usually, it is obvious who should be first author, but confusion and conflict can occur when several people are working on a project. The research group should resolve who is going to be first author long before it is time to write the paper so that if there is any jockeying for position, it occurs early and is resolved. It also means that the other co-authors can scale back their investment in the project and allow the first author to lead. If first-authorship is not resolved early, several people may all feel they have made the largest contribution to a project. Sometimes, even if a first author is decided early, another person contributes as much, and in that case two people can share first authorship. This often happens when one person did most of the work but left the lab and someone else finished the project and wrote the paper. Shared first authorship is usually indicated with an asterisk after the last names of the first two authors on the title page and a footnote indicating "Dr. A and Dr. B contributed equally to the work." If you have such a paper on your CV, you should indicate shared first authorship in the same way.

Who should be last author? The last author is usually the senior author (the terms are used interchangeably) and is responsible for the overall conduct of the study, including its accuracy and ethical components. The last author assumes overall responsibility for the paper; in other words, "the buck stops here." The last author is often also the person who obtained funding to do the study. Traditionally, the last author was also the corresponding author, and the two terms were synonymous, but this is no longer the case.

Who is the corresponding author? The corresponding author is the person who communicates with the journal during submission, peer review, revision, review of proofs, and publication. The corresponding author is also the person who submits the paper electronically and ensures that all the authors complete the conflict of interest and copyright transfer forms. In the old days you could submit a paper by mailing a cover letter and 3 copies of the manuscript to the journal; now someone has to spend several hours filling out electronic forms. As a result, senior authors often delegate the task and are seldom also corresponding authors; thus, the terms are no longer synonymous.

Why does authorship matter? You might wonder why people make such a fuss over authorship. Authorship matters because it is a quantifiable measure of your scientific productivity and impact, and it is a public acknowledgement of your contributions. Promotion committees (Chapter 20) use an individual's publication record to make decisions about promotion. In some countries this is formalized; for example, you need x publications as first author in a journal with an impact factor above y to be promoted. In other countries, committees use a less formal gestalt of your publication record. For these reasons, authorship is valuable. An investigation published in *Science* (2) that described the existence of a market for scientific authorship in China illustrates this value. Individuals could purchase authorship for a fee ranging from $1600 to $26,300; authorship on articles in journals listed in the Science Citation Index was the most expensive.

Why does first or last authorship matter? You might also wonder why people get exercised about the order of the authors. One reason is that first and last authorship are particularly valued by promotion committees. If your name is hidden in the middle of a bunch of authors, the importance of your scientific contribution is unclear, and you could have contributed very little. For example, you will see papers, particularly in the genetics area, with hundreds of authors who clearly contributed little to the actual paper. However, if you are first author, yours was the most important contribution, and you are accorded primary ownership of the work. Last authorship is a sign of scientific independence and maturity and the ability to envision, fund, and direct a project.

What about middle authors? Except for the last author, the order is usually determined by how much each person contributed to the paper. For the first few names (perhaps the first 3 to 6) the order has some implications. For example, the second author is thought to have contributed substantially more than the seventh author. Also, sometimes in large multicenter trials there are too many authors to list and approximately six names are listed as "writing for the ABC Research Study Group." Clearly, it is more prestigious to have your name on the cover of the journal than buried in an appendix of contributing authors. In addition to each individual's contribution, the order of authors is also affected by human nature; some authors jockey for position because they are more aggressive or self-centered. Generally, other than first, second, and last authorship, I don't think order is worth fussing about.

The title page – Short Title, Word Count, Correspondence: The short title is used as a header on alternate pages in the published manuscript and should tell the reader what the paper is about. The word count tells the editor how long your paper is, and if the journal restricts the length of papers, that you are within the limits. The address for correspondence provides the contact information for the corresponding author.

2) Abstract

The abstract is the only section most readers look at: The abstract is important because it is the only part of your paper most people read, and because reviewers have often made a gut decision about your paper after reading it. The abstract should summarize the question (why), methods (how), results (what you found), and conclusion. I find it helpful to use a structured abstract with the following headings: Introduction, Methods, Results, and Conclusion. This structure makes it easy to see how your abstract is weighted. If the Introduction occupies 10 lines of a 20 line abstract, the weight is poorly distributed.

Be specific in the abstract: Include numbers, measures of spread (e.g., standard deviation or confidence intervals), and P values to support the major findings in the abstract. Which of the following two sentences do you find most helpful? *There was a highly significant difference in CD4 count between patients with HIV who received beetroot compared to those who did not.* Or, *There was a highly significant difference in CD4 count (32 ± 150 cells, P=0.096) between patients with HIV who received beetroot (n=4) compared to those who did not (n=3).* You can see that without numbers the statement is opinion rather than fact; with numbers it is obvious that there is no clinical or statistical significance.

3) Introduction

If haven't hooked the reader after the Introduction you have lost the game: The point of the Introduction is to sell the idea, not to review the world literature. The format is usually context, problem, and quest for a solution. The context paragraphs give readers the background information they need to understand why the problem is important. The problem section tells readers what the major unanswered question (the knowledge gap) is. The solution/quest section tells readers how you can answer the question (solution) or work towards a solution (quest). The Introduction tells the reader why you did the study, and to do that effectively, you use the extant literature as a frame to define what is not known (i.e., the knowledge gap). You must also convince the reader that filling the knowledge gap (i.e., answering the question) is vitally important. After the Introduction you want the reader to think: *that is an interesting question and it is important to know the answer.* On the other hand, if the reader thinks: *we already know the answer* (not new); or, *so what if we know the answer* (unimportant); or, *I don't understand why they did the study* (your rationale is unclear), you have lost the game. The benefit of an interesting and important knowledge gap is that you do not have to find a positive outcome; readers will appreciate the significance of the answer, whether it is positive or negative.

Keep the Introduction short and focused: A common mistake is to begin a paper by trying to summarize the literature comprehensively. Rather, your Introduction should draw on the literature to explain briefly and clearly why you did the study (knowledge gap) and why the question is important. A single double spaced page is often enough. If you have more than two pages of Introduction, it is too long.

4) Methods

What you did and how you did it: The Methods section is straightforward and describes what you did and how you did it. I write the Methods while I am doing the study because the procedures are fresh in my mind. Ideally, the Methods should be detailed enough that an informed investigator can reproduce your study. You can't always do this because of word count limitations. An online supplementary appendix can be helpful. Make sure you describe your sample size calculation and statistical analysis. It is also important to say that your study was approved by the appropriate human or animal ethical oversight committees.

5) Results

What you found: The Results section describes what you found, not your opinion of what you found. In clinical papers there is never any interpretation in the Results; in basic science papers authors sometimes interpret the results of one experiment to provide the rationale for the results of the next one. When you write the Results, you do not have to include every piece of data. It is painful when someone does a study as part of a thesis and submits a paper that has a dozen data tables, many irrelevant to the story. The aim of the thesis was to show the examiners your exquisite attention to scientific method; the aim of the paper is to tell a story. Make sure that the important results (i.e., those that address your primary hypothesis) feature prominently in the Results.

Use subheadings to organize the Results: It is useful to have subheadings for the different sections of the Results. Some journals frown on such subheadings, but even if you eventually delete them, they help organize your results. For example, the following subheadings provide a clear outline for the results of a study: *Study Population; Effect of Beetroot on Insulin Sensitivity; Effect of Beetroot on Vascular Response; Relationship between Change in Insulin Sensitivity and Vascular Response; Adherence and Side Effects.*

Results should not duplicate Tables: Generally, the Results section should not duplicate too much information that is in tables and figures. For example, in most clinical papers Table 1 shows the characteristics of the study groups and includes numbers that summarize their age, race, sex, and other characteristics; this information should not be duplicated in the text. So in the Results you should not write, *"The average age of the patients was 25.2 ± 3.2 years and of controls 24.9 ± 3.1 years (p=0.52; 46.4% of patients and 47.5 % of controls were women were women....)"* and so on if those numbers are already in Table 1. Rather, tell the story, *"The patient and control groups were well matched for age and sex.... (Table 1)."* Some duplication of numbers text and tables is inevitable, but don't overdo it.

6) Discussion

Tell a story: The Discussion, like the Introduction, is not a literature review. The purpose of the Discussion is to put your findings into context and tell the reader what they mean. I like to state the most important new findings in first paragraph of the Discussion. Then, you tell a story that shows where your findings fit into current knowledge, how they add to it, what they mean, what their implications are for clinical care or other research, and the limitations of your study.

Avoid bias: You have probably discussed a movie with someone and from their description you can hardly believe you saw the same movie. Sometimes I get that feeling when I read the Discussion section of a paper, and the authors have built castles on the flimsiest results or are so wedded to their hypothesis that they maintain it is true despite lack of statistical significance. Unlike a movie, you and the reader are both working from the same set of data, so restrain your imagination and base your discussion on the facts.

P=0.051 is not statistically significant: Statisticians shake their heads at our obsession with P value cutoffs that dichotomize the outcome of a study; indeed, there is no material difference between P=0.049 and P=0.051. However, if your Methods declare, *P values <0.05 were considered statistically significant*, then P=0.051 is not significant (by your own definition). You can do all kinds of things such as discussing sample size, statistical power, confidence intervals,

Bayesian approaches, future studies, biological plausibility, and so on, but what you cannot do is pretend no one has noticed that 0.051 is >0.05 and discuss the finding as though it is statistically significant. I have chosen the finest line of P=0.051 to illustrate the point, but you will come across many papers that build castles on outcomes with much larger P values as if they were significant.

No Results in Discussion: A common mistake is to repeat results in the Discussion section. You have already presented the results; your job now is to interpret them. Another common mistake is to present new results in the Discussion for the first time. For example, to check that your major finding was not confounded, you say you performed some additional sensitivity analyses adjusting for potentially confounding covariates and give the results. The place to present those additional analyses is in the Results; the place to discuss them is the Discussion.

Your limitations paragraph need not blow your foot off: Towards the end of the Discussion it is usual to have a paragraph about the limitations of your study. This is not a place to shoot yourself in the foot. All studies have strengths and offsetting limitations, so instead of: *Our study was small and underpowered*, offset the limitations with some strengths: *Our study was small, but the homogeneous group of patients studied allowed us detect a significant difference in....*

Conclusion – stick to the data: Traditionally, the last paragraph of the Discussion is the conclusion. You briefly (in one or two sentences) summarize the major finding of your paper. Most editors insist that you base the conclusion only on data that are in the paper. For example, we found that coronary artery calcification scores were high in patients with rheumatoid arthritis. A reasonable conclusion would be: *In conclusion, coronary artery calcification scores, a recognized marker of coronary atherosclerosis, were higher in patients with RA than controls.* A highly speculative conclusion would be: *In conclusion, ischemic heart disease is more common in patients with RA and measurement of coronary artery calcification may allow the identification of high-risk patients for targeted interventions such as aggressive anti-inflammatory therapy.* The second conclusion may sound reasonable, but we did not characterize ischemic heart disease, nor did we show that coronary artery calcification scores identify a high-risk subgroup, nor did we study the effect of anti-inflammatory therapy on cardiovascular outcomes.

7) Acknowledgements, conflict of interest, and funding sources

Do not acknowledge your grade school English teacher (mentor Alastair Wood)**:** The Acknowledgements section, if needed, is brief and thanks individuals who contributed directly to the paper but are not authors. For example, *We thank Jane Smith, PhD who performed the catecholamine assays.* Many journals require you to obtain permission from the people you acknowledge. One reason they do this is to allow people who are acknowledged to claim authorship if they believe they should be authors. Another reason is to prevent authors from using the acknowledgements section for name dropping. For example, your paper would seem much more important if you acknowledge a Nobel Prize winner for "invaluable advice."

Pay attention to conflict of interest: Some journals ask you to include statements about funding and conflict of interest on the title page rather than at the end of the manuscript. List the authors' conflicts of interest as requested by the journal. Most journals request only financial conflicts of interest. Remember, it is the appearance of a conflict of interest that is important, not whether you think there was an actual conflict of interest (Chapter 27). Pay attention to the details; it will be embarrassing if you declared no conflicts of interest and are later called to task in the correspondence columns of the journal or in the newspapers for deceiving readers.

List all funding sources: List all the funding sources that supported the work and the people who performed the study. If you are supported by grants from NIH, it is important to cite them. If you cite a grant, it means that the publication can be included in the progress report for that grant. The work in most papers is supported by several grants; cite them all. If you received support from industry, acknowledge that and ensure that your conflict of interest statement is complete.

8) References

Formatting references: Each journal has a particular reference format. Some have superscript numbers in the text[1,2] and list the references in numeric order.

1. Brown AB, Green J. Referencing for medical journals. J Ref 2002;100;1-4.
2. Azure A, Green J. Superscript is superior. J Med Ref 2004;400; 123-5.

Others use names in the text (Brown AB, 2002; Azure A 2004) and then list the references alphabetically.

Azure A, Green J. Superscript is superior. J Med Ref 2004;400; 123-5.
Brown AB, Green J. Referencing for medical journals. J Ref 2002;100;1-4.

The ICMJE recommends uniform guidelines for the formatting of references (3), but journals have endless style permutations. It is a waste of time to retype and renumber references manually. Use a program to manage your references; commonly used programs are Reference Manager (support discontinued 2016) and EndNote, but there are several available, including some that are free (4). Initially, I used a separate file of references for each paper, but I soon learnt it was easier to keep one large file (it now has more than 5,000 references).

Limit the number of references cited and choose carefully: Some journals limit the number of references you can cite. Even if a journal does not mention a maximum, limit yourself to 30-40 references, unless you are writing a review article. Select the papers you cite so that they support statements that are crucial to your argument. Where possible, cite the paper that made the original observation, except when the observation has already entered common wisdom (e.g., hypertension is associated with increased risk of stroke; obesity is a common cause of morbidity). Generally, if you have a choice between equally appropriate references, cite the higher quality papers.

Cite the reference that scooped you: If you have been scooped, cite the paper that scooped you rather than pretend you don't know about it. When editors search for reviewers and when reviewers search for information they will find the paper that you would rather ignore, so it is better to acknowledge the paper and find reasons it strengthened rather than weakened the burning need to perform your study.

Self-citation – be judicious: If you don't think your own work is important enough to cite, why should anyone else cite it? On the other hand, if 20 of the 30 references you cite are to your own work, there are two possible interpretations. First, no one else in the world is particularly interested in this area. Second, your sense of self-importance needs calibration. Neither interpretation is good for your paper.

9) Tables and Figures

Have a reasonable number of high quality Tables and Figures: More is not always better. Some journals limit the number of Tables and Figures to a total of five. For clinical journals, resist the temptation to combine several figures into one with many panels. For basic science journals, this approach is the norm and leads to extraordinarily complex figures that are difficult to understand.

Use big text in labels: When the journal shrinks a figure for publication, the text of the X and Y-axis labels also shrinks. A common mistake is to use a font size for axes labels that looks reasonable in the manuscript you submit but looks puny when the figure is shrunk for publication.

Include measures of spread: A figure that summarizes data without a measure of spread such as standard deviation or 95% confidence interval cannot be interpreted.

What is the message of your figure? Many people believe that the purpose of a figure is to summarize data visually. To some extent that is true. But the real purpose of a figure is to convey a message. The message is often simple (e.g., groups A and B look different, or groups C and D do not look different). You have a problem if the reader looks at your figure and questions the message. If your figure is trying to send the message that two groups are different, then they should look different. Conversely, if the difference is not statistically significant, the figure should not look as if the groups could be different. High-impact papers often have a "T-shirt figure" (mentor Alastair Wood) – a figure that, if you reproduced it on your T-shirt, would convey the message and its importance in a way that everyone understands, unequivocally and instantly.

10) Table and Figure legends

Tables and Figures should be able to stand alone. In other words, if you looked at just the Figures or Tables, you should be able to understand them completely. You should explain all abbreviations in the footnotes (even if you already explained them in the text).

Summary

1. Give thought to your title.

2. Use the ICMJE criteria for authorship.

3. Use a structured abstract and include numbers and P values.

4. The point of the Introduction is to sell the idea, not to review the literature. Keep the Introduction brief.

5. The point of the Discussion is to tell readers what your findings mean, not to review the literature.

6. Tables should not repeat a lot of the Results text.

7. The point of a Figure is to make a point.

8. Tables and Figures should be self-standing.

9. Tell a story.

Resources

1. International Committee of Medical Journal Editors. Sponsorship, authorship and accountability. Recommendations for the conduct, reporting, editing and publication of scholarly work in medical journals. www.icmje.org.

2. Hvistendahl M. China's publication bazaar. *Science* 2013:342;1035-1039.

3. The ICMJE uniform guidelines for the formatting of references http://www.nlm.nih.gov/bsd/uniform_requirements.html

4. Some reference management software. https://en.wikipedia.org/wiki/Comparison_of_reference_management_software

5. Strange K. Authorship: why not just toss a coin? Am J Physiol Cell Physiol 2008:295;C567-C575.

6. Sismondo S. Ghost management: How much of the medical literature is shaped behind the scenes by the pharmaceutical industry? PLOS Medicine 2007:4; 1429-1433.

7. Ross JS, Hill KP, Eligman DS, Krumholz HM. Guest authorship and ghostwriting in publications related to rofecoxib. A case study of industry documents from rofecoxib litigation. JAMA 2008:299;1800-12.

8. Kyriacou DN. The enduring evolution of the P Value. JAMA 2016:315:1113-5.

Chapter 8
Writing a paper – how to write and submit it

The most important sentence in the paper

Which is the most important sentence of the paper? Good suggestions are the first and last sentences of the Introduction, the last sentence of the Conclusion, and the title. They are all indeed important, but a paper (and a grant) is like an ice-dance – every move (sentence) must be at least respectable and preferably outstanding, and the most important move is the one in which the judges see you make a mistake and fall. Mistakes include clichés, unnecessary complexity, illegible figures, breaks in logic, selective literature citation, a poor question, poor methods, and grammatical errors. This chapter is not a grammar primer, nor is it a comprehensive manual for scientific writing, it only provides direction.

What you have to say and how you say it are both important

Perfect writing cannot compensate for a poor study; however, poor writing can sink a good study. The secrets to good writing are effort, attention to every word, telling a story, and obsessive revising. Writing is fundamental to an academic scientific career; if you cannot learn to write competently or do not enjoy it, this may not be the career for you. With hard work and practice, most people can learn to be passable scientific writers.

Perspiration is more important than inspiration

A few people are born writers; most of us struggle. Writing a paper is laborious, and if you wait for inspiration, or a block of uninterrupted time, your paper will never be written. Use your time management skills (Chapter 6) to make blocks of time, and then write your paper, one paragraph at a time. Write the Introduction section before you do a single experiment. Unless you can frame an interesting and important question, you do not have a study that is worth doing. Write the Methods section while you are doing the studies. Once you have finished the studies and analyzed the data, construct the key Tables and Figures. After that, the rest of the paper falls into place naturally.

Paragraphs headings frame your story

We use words, sentences, and paragraphs to build a story. Just as a builder first frames a house, it is helpful to construct a frame for your story by using paragraph headings that summarize the key message of each paragraph. If you read just the paragraph headings, you can follow the story. For example, here are paragraph headings for the Introduction section of a paper we wrote about a study of cholesterol efflux in patients with rheumatoid arthritis (RA).

1. RA is a common disease and has increased cardiovascular risk.
2. Cardiovascular risk factors identified in the general population do not explain the increased risk in RA.
3. HDL is an important cardiovascular risk factor but concentrations are not altered in RA.
4. HDL decreases cardiovascular risk through several mechanisms, including HDL-mediated cholesterol efflux, and these are poorly related to HDL concentrations,
5. HDL-mediated cholesterol efflux may predict risk better than HDL concentrations.
6. The relationship between HDL-mediated cholesterol efflux and cardiovascular risk in RA is unknown (knowledge gap) and might explain increased risk in RA (importance).

You can see how the paragraph headings, even without any additional text, frame the story. The content of the headings will be incorporated into each paragraph so that you can eventually delete them before you submit the paper. For grants (Chapter 12), I keep brief headings (as done in this book).

Keep paragraphs on point

You will see from the previous example that each paragraph heading is about a small, defined idea or topic. In fact, the first sentence of the paragraph will often paraphrase the entire paragraph and is sometimes called the "topic sentence" because it tells the reader what the paragraph is about. While you are writing, these headings delineate the paragraph topic and prevent your thoughts and writing from wandering into other interesting but off-topic areas.

Keep paragraphs short

Long paragraphs make it difficult for a reader to follow your story. If you have a paragraph that is longer than 8 lines, it is likely that your writing has strayed beyond a single concept and that you should have started a new paragraph for a new topic.

Sentences are the building blocks for each paragraph

Each paragraph starts with a sentence that frames its topic. Short, simple sentences are easy to understand. Also, sentences that have the subject and verb close together at the beginning of the sentence are easy to understand. Sentences must be linked to tell a story. Logic links them; for example, you can use a concept from the previous sentence to introduce the next sentence. They are also linked by words that facilitate transition and narrative (e.g., although, however, moreover, previously, nevertheless, also, besides, furthermore, therefore, thus, finally, in fact, recently, for example, in other words, because).

et al, et al, et al

A common beginner's mistake is to present the findings of different studies as a shopping list of et als. This suggests you can't be bothered to craft a coherent story. For example: *It has been shown by Smith et al. that rheumatoid arthritis (RA) was associated with hypertension. Jones et al. reported that RA was not associated with hypertension. Green et al. indicated that hypertension was associated with endothelial dysfunction in RA, but White et al. reported conflicting findings. We studied the relationship between endothelial function and hypertension in RA.*

With a little thought we can rewrite the paragraph and tell a logical story using ideas and words that link sentences. We can also improve the writing by eliminating unnecessary words. For example: *The prevalence of hypertension was increased in patients with active rheumatoid arthritis (RA) (Smith) but not in those with well-controlled disease (Jones). Similarly, endothelial dysfunction, a precursor of hypertension, was present in patients with active RA (Green) but improved with control of inflammation (White). Thus, we examined the hypothesis that inflammation, by causing endothelial dysfunction, is a reversible mechanism underlying hypertension in RA.*

Revise, revise, revise

Revision and rewriting are time-consuming, painful, and essential. Revision involves deconstructing each sentence to eliminate errors and unnecessary words and ensure logical flow. I number the drafts of a paper and often proceed through 20 or more versions before submission. There are no shortcuts.

Learn to write with your mentor

Mentors have different approaches to writing a paper with a trainee. As a mentor, I like to see the paper at a relatively early stage when the paragraph headings are mapped out and the data tables constructed so that I can direct the big picture. Then, unless there are problems or questions about direction, I prefer not to work on the paper until the trainee feels it is in excellent shape. From a mentor's point of view, it is frustrating to work on many successive early rough drafts of the paper, each with many obvious errors that the mentee should have corrected.

Your mentor is likely to rewrite your paper

My mentor preferred to edit a paper version of the manuscript with a red pen, a pair of scissors, and sticky tape. Initially, I was horrified to receive my papers back with more handwritten red ink than printed text and with pieces of paper cut out, moved, or added. When you get a version of the paper that has more changes than original text, don't take it personally. Mentors treat their own manuscripts the same way – the first draft always stinks, no matter who wrote it. But it is important to understand why your mentor made particular changes. When I typed my mentor's handwritten changes into my electronic version of the manuscript I could see why the changes improved the paper. These days it is easy (but not as educational) to electronically "accept all changes."

Make sure that you and your mentor are working on the same version

Make sure everyone knows who has the "live" version of the manuscript. If your mentor has the paper for editing, make sure it is the most recent version. Also, don't make changes to the paper until you receive the "live" version back. It will irritate your mentor to work on the paper and find that you have been working on the same version, introducing new errors into sections that he or she just edited. If your mentor is taking too long to edit a paper, a diplomatic nudge is in order: "When do you think I can get the paper back from you, I'd like to work on the…."

Your mentor is not infallible but don't sneak your changes back

Don't be shy about correcting your mentor's text. Your mentor can make spelling and grammatical errors and may not know the data or relevant literature as well as you do. Make your edits in track changes and explain with a comment if need be. But don't put your version back into the edited paper without showing that you have done so and providing an explanation. It is irritating for a mentor to make the same corrections to subsequent drafts of the paper. If you disagree or don't understand some of the changes, discuss them.

Soliciting comments from co-authors

Once you and your mentor are happy with a version that is almost ready for submission, send the paper to all the co-authors. It is useful to provide them with a time-line. For example: *We would like to submit at the end of the month so if you could please get your comments to me by the 15th that would be great.* It also means that on the 16th you can send a reminder. It is ironic that the people who contributed least are often the slowest to respond.

Dealing with comments from co-authors

Don't automatically make every change a co-author suggests. If a co-author asks a specific question, you should answer it – but not necessarily change the manuscript. One approach is to correct the errors co-authors spot, clarify sections they found confusing, and discuss the remaining changes with your mentor. Once you and your mentor have made the changes that you think improve the paper, circulate the final version to all co-authors. Some co-authors get offended if the changes they suggested are not implemented. Therefore, when you circulate the final version, say that your mentor decided on the changes (a statement that should be true). Unless the changes were extensive, the time-line for commenting on the final version can be much shorter. For example: *Dear Co-Authors, Attached please find the final version of the manuscript. Dr. Jones and I have incorporated many of the changes everyone suggested. The version attached is very similar to the one you previously reviewed in detail. We would like to submit at the end of the week. If you could review it before then and let me know if there are any errors, I would be grateful. If I don't hear from you by Thursday evening, I will submit on Friday. Best, Mary.*

Choosing a target journal – impact factor

Your mentor will help choose an appropriate target journal. Although you can see articles in journals that are not indexed in PubMed through other search engines, they are largely invisible to most of your audience. So, make sure that the journal is indexed in PubMed. Another consideration is the journal's impact factor. Although people criticize the impact factor as being a poor measure of quality, the higher the impact factor the more prominent the journal. The impact factor for each journal listed in Journal Citation Reports® (Thomson Reuters) is calculated annually by dividing how often articles published in the journal in the previous 2 years were cited during a particular year by the total number of papers published in the 2 years. For example, if a journal published 90 articles in 2014 and 110 in 2015 and these were cited 400 times in 2016, then the 2016 impact factor is 2.0 (i.e., 400 citations divided by (90+110) articles). Obviously, the 2016 impact factors are only available midway through 2017. Journals with an impact factor higher than 10 (approximately 180 of 8500 journals listed in Journal Citation Reports®) are sometimes considered high impact.

To give you a sense of the variation, here are the approximate 2016 impact factors from Journal Citation Reports® (Thomson Reuters) for a few journals: *New England Journal of Medicine 72, Lancet 48, JAMA 44, Nature 40, Nature Medicine 30, Circulation 19, Annals of Internal Medicine 17, Journal of Clinical Investigation 13, Blood 13, Hypertension 7, Chest 6, Journal of Biological Chemistry 4,* and *Plos One* 3.

Where to publish – your career

Ideally, you would like to publish research in a journal that your grant reviewers as well as your clinical peers read and respect. But sometimes these two target audiences are not congruent. For example, an endocrinologist performing cardiovascular research funded by the National Heart, Lung, and Blood Institute (NHLBI), may have to choose between publishing in cardiovascular journals (familiar to grant reviewers) or endocrinology journals (read by clinical peers).

Where to publish – aim high?

If you never submit your work to high-impact journals you will never publish in them. On the other hand, high-impact journals reject the overwhelming majority of the papers they receive. You might think that you have nothing to lose by submitting your paper to a high-impact journal. Other than waiting approximately 6-8 weeks for the reviews (or a few days if the editors triage it), what do you have to lose? Unfortunately, each time a journal rejects your paper you receive a metaphorical kick in the stomach. It does not matter that you were fairly sure the high-impact journal paper would reject your paper, your morale and that of your group suffers. If several journals reject your paper, even though they were high-impact and you didn't really expect them to accept the paper, you feel that your work is worthless.

Where to publish – aim low?

Why would you ever target a journal with an impact factor and reputation lower than you believe appropriate for your paper? The usual answer is that you need to publish the paper quickly and cannot afford the time it takes for a more prestigious journal to review and potentially reject it. If you need to publish a paper quickly, it is usually because you think someone is about to scoop you, or you need to publish the paper before you submit a grant.

Where to publish – avoid low quality journals

Low quality online-only journals have proliferated. Once you have published a few papers, your email address will be public, and obscure journals that are money-making ventures inundate you with requests to join editorial boards and submit papers; some call them predatory journals (1,2). It is hard to identify these journals because their names are often very similar to those of reputable journals. If a journal is not indexed in PubMed, avoid it. Online sites provide opinions about potentially problematic journals (2).

When to publish

There is a tension between publishing frequently in medium to low-impact journals and publishing less frequently in high-impact journals. It is wise to diversify your portfolio and do both. The danger of focusing exclusively on high-impact papers is that they are not just an agglomeration of medium-impact work; you cannot guarantee a high-impact publication no matter how much data you collect. High-impact papers are the confluence of luck, creativity, and hard work. You could spend three years preparing a high-impact paper only to have it rejected and end up in a medium-impact journal, leaving you with a CV that suggests low productivity. Despite what many people say, the number of papers you have published does matter for promotion (Chapter 20). But it is not all about numbers, the quality of your papers also matters. It is difficult to measure the quality of a paper. Purists say that it does not matter where you publish a paper because an expert scientist can judge the quality of the science independently. In reality, people use the impact factor of the journal and the number of times your paper is cited by others as surrogates for quality. Aim for a solid publication record that shows productivity and includes some publications in high-impact journals.

Plan publishable units but avoid salami

You could work forever to perform the perfect study and publish nothing (mentor Alastair Wood). To avoid this, plan your work with goals that lead to a paper. Planning your work in publishable units is helpful because publications are one metric by which your productivity is judged when you apply for grants and for promotion. Fascinating work that is never published cannot sustain you. However, salami publication (discussed later under responsible authorship) and chopping your work into "least publishable units" (3) is bad and will be obvious when someone looks at your CV.

Should you contact the editor before submitting your paper?

If you are writing a review article or an opinion piece, you might want to ask the editor if the journal is interested in your piece before you submit. Original articles, on the other hand, are accepted or rejected based on scientific priority and it is difficult to think of an appropriate pre-submission question for the editor other than whether the paper is suitable for the journal. You should not need to the editor to tell you that. Some journals mandate editorial pre-review, but that is part of their triage process.

The positive and negative sides of a presubmission enquiry

A positive effect of an unsolicited presubmission enquiry is that you might communicate with a particular friendly associate editor and could then subsequently ask for your paper to be assigned to that person. However, you can request a particular associate editor in your cover letter without a presubmisson enquiry. A potential negative effect of a presubmission enquiry is that the journal thinks you are trying to schmooze and game the system. When I was an editor, some authors would send their abstract (or even the entire paper) and ask whether the journal would be interested in the work. My gut reaction was that if the authors were seasoned professionals they would know if their paper was suitable for the journal, and that the request was a disguised attempt to build rapport and influence the process. For original articles, avoid a presubmission enquiry unless the journal requires it. For unsolicited review articles, a presubmission enquiry is useful.

A presubmission solicitation does not guarantee acceptance

An editor might leave a card on your poster at a meeting asking you to submit the full paper to that journal. If you look around, you will see the same card on several posters. Editors solicit business for their journals, and the invitation to submit is not a guarantee of acceptance (or even of great interest), although it will make rejection by that journal rankle more than usual. Similarly, if a journal solicits a review article, there is no guarantee that it will be accepted – although most usually are.

Suggesting potential reviewers

Many journals ask you to suggest potential reviewers. You obviously cannot suggest people who have a conflict of interest. I usually leave the "suggested reviewers" section blank, but if you are obliged to provide names, then suggest people with expertise in the area. You do not have to know the people you suggest; you can select potential reviewers and obtain their email addresses from PubMed. You can suggest people who know you peripherally, but don't choose them because you think they will give you an easy ride; your acquaintances can be your harshest critics.

Avoiding potential reviewers

Some journals ask if there are individuals you prefer not to review your paper, and even if the journal does not ask, you can make the request in your cover letter. Generally, you should use this option sparingly and only to avoid reviewers that you believe have a scientific or personal conflict of interest.

The cover letter

Most journals ask you to submit a cover letter, but for some it is not obligatory. Your cover letter should be brief (less than a page) and focus on why the paper is new and important. In other words, you are trying to sell your paper. The editor will read your abstract and likely your paper; therefore, you do not need to repeat extensive details about the paper in your cover letter.

Make sure you address your cover letter to the correct editor and journal (not to the editor of the journal that previously rejected the paper). Address the editor by name; do not use a generic salutation such as "Dear Editor."

The Instructions to Authors section for each journal is different. Follow the instructions. Some journals ask for specific information in the cover letter – usually that all authors qualify for authorship, that the work is original and has not been submitted elsewhere, and a list of other publications that have derived from the work. An example of a cover letter follows.

Dear Dr. Smith,

I would be grateful if you would consider the enclosed paper: "*Increased Coronary-Artery Atherosclerosis in Rheumatoid Arthritis: Relationship with Disease Duration and Cardiovascular Risk Factors*" for publication in the Journal of Cardiovascular Rheumatology as an original article.

We show for the first time that that the prevalence and severity of coronary atherosclerosis is increased in patients with rheumatoid arthritis. This information is of general interest and importance not only because rheumatoid arthritis is a common disease but also because it is associated with a 2-fold increased prevalence of coronary heart disease. This paper is also important because it defines the relationship between inflammation and atherosclerosis. Furthermore, the fact that atherosclerosis was not increased in patients with early rheumatoid arthritis suggests that there is a window of time in which to intervene. Thus, our findings have the potential to change the way cardiovascular risk is assessed and treated in patients with inflammatory diseases.

All the authors have approved the final version of the manuscript for submission and qualify for authorship. The work has not been published elsewhere and is not under consideration by another journal.

Thank you very much for your consideration.

Yours sincerely,

Before you hit send

A sloppy paper is a poor vehicle for your work. Before you hit send, make sure that there are no typos, that you have submitted the correct version of the paper, and that "track changes" and co-authors' comments are not visible or embedded in the manuscript.

Responsible conduct of research and authorship

In addition to the criteria for authorship, several other aspects of responsible conduct of research (Chapter 27) are important in scientific publishing.

Plagiarism: Plagiarism is passing another person's ideas or words off as your own. You cannot copy from someone else's work unless you use quotation marks and tell the reader where the citation comes from. You can imagine how you might plagiarize text accidentally if you cut and paste text from another document into your own work (planning to use the text as a reminder to yourself to write something) and then later forget that you did not write that text. Never copy or cut and paste from the work of others. Even if you do so from your own work, it would be self-plagiarism.

Plagiarism of ideas is more subtle than plagiarism of text and can be deliberate. For example, someone who reviews a paper could deliberately take ideas or methods from the paper and apply them. Or, someone who reads about a neat hypothesis that explains their findings could deliberately raise the hypothesis in their paper without citing the person whose idea it was. Pay scrupulous attention to citing others appropriately. Plagiarism can also be inadvertent.

Cryptomnesia or inadvertent plagiarism: We are all at risk for committing plagiarism unconsciously. For example, I review a paper and a few months later, long after I have forgotten the paper, an idea from the paper percolates up in my thoughts but now as my own brilliant idea. This phenomenon is termed cryptomnesia – a forgotten idea surfacing as a new idea. In science, problems occur when a scientist who has heard an idea from someone else claims to have come up with the idea spontaneously. Science is built on the work of others and we often don't know who had a particular idea first, but make sure you attribute ideas in your own work to their sources.

Studies show that people often take credit for an idea that was not their own – particularly if they think they have improved it. In my experience, more senior investigators are the worst culprits – perhaps because so many ideas cross their desks, perhaps because any one idea among many is not critical to their careers, or perhaps because they believe that the advancement of science trumps minor details such as appropriate allocation of credit. In a novel, *The Cheese Monkey*, by Chipp Kid, an art student, is angry that a friend has stolen his idea. The friend replies: "I didn't *steal* it! You left that idea squealing on my doorstep." Once you release an idea publicly it is free for anyone to take, so think before you talk about ideas you might want to take further.

Fabrication: Fabrication of data accounts for the most egregious cases of research misconduct. More subtle, and harder to discover, are changing a few numbers to move the P-value in the desired direction and editing figures to "improve" them. Such behavior is dishonest and unethical and has serious consequences.

Simultaneous submission: You must not submit the same manuscript to more than one journal simultaneously. You might rationalize that you will save time and can always withdraw from one journal if both accept your paper. However, simultaneous submission exploits the goodwill and resources of journals and reviewers, and is unethical.

Salami publication: It is often acceptable to use the same set of patients to publish several papers that address different questions (e.g., the many papers from the Framingham study). It is unacceptable to use the same set of patients to publish several papers that provide minimally incremental information – salami publication. For example, it would be hard to justify the need for the following set of publications that used the same data: Pharmacokinetics of X; Pharmacodynamics of X; Pharmacokinetic modeling of X, Pharmacokinetic and pharmacodynamic modeling of X, and so on. When you submit a paper that includes published data, you should reference those papers and explain the overlap to the reader (in the paper) and to the editor (in the cover letter) and describe how the current paper addresses a new question.

Duplicate and redundant publication: Duplicate publication is when the same paper is published in two different journals. There is no justification for doing this. The fact that the two journals are in different languages, have different audiences, or exist on different continents is not a justification. Redundant publication is when essentially the same data and ideas are published with minor modifications (e.g., an extra handful of patients) and often with different authors. Duplicate and redundant publications occur because authors do not tell editors and readers what they have done, nor do they refer to the other publication and reference it. Duplicate and redundant publication will lead to retraction of articles and public censure.

What happens after you have submitted your paper?

After you have submitted your paper, you will usually receive an automated notification. Editorial staff screen incoming papers, and if a paper is unsuitable for the journal (e.g., an original publication is submitted to a journal that only publishes reviews), they notify authors immediately. For many journals an associate editor or other members of the editorial team triage papers before sending some out for review. If they think the journal is unlikely to publish the paper (for reasons of novelty, importance, interest, validity) they reject it without external review, usually within a week. If a week goes by and you have heard nothing, you can usually assume that the journal has sent your paper to external reviewers. You can track your manuscript and see if it is "out for review" or "awaiting an editorial decision" on the websites of most journals.

How soon can I expect a decision?

You can expect a decision within 8-12 weeks, usually sooner. If 12 weeks pass and you have heard nothing, you might feel like prodding the editorial office. But the remedy for a slow decision is patience. It is difficult for the editorial office to lose track of papers because most journals use an electronic manuscript management system. So the editor responsible for your paper is almost certainly already receiving frequent automated emails saying that the decision on your manuscript is seriously overdue. The usual problem is that one reviewer is late or has reneged. The risk of prodding editors is that the quickest way for them to solve the problem is to reject the paper (mentor Alastair Wood). It is never a good idea to call the editor about a slow review.

The decision

The reviewers submit their reviews to the editorial office and an editor reads them, looks at your paper again, and makes a decision. The decision is based on what the reviewers say, what the editor thinks of the paper, what the journal needs, and all the other variables that influence subjective human decisions. You will then receive an email that almost certainly says something like this: *Dear Dr. X, I regret to inform you that we are unable to accept your paper for publication....* The next chapter talks about your response to the different varieties of this email.

Summary

1. Writing is hard work and improves with practice.

2. Use paragraph headings to frame your story.

3. Keep your paragraphs short.

4. Learn to write.

5. Be a responsible writer.

6. Choose an appropriate target journal.

7. Pay attention to detail.

Resources

1. Shen C, Björk BC. 'Predatory' open access: a longitudinal study of article volumes and market characteristics. BMC Med. 2015 Oct 1;13:230. PMID: 26423063; PMC4589914.

2. An archived list of journals considered by some to be potentially problematic. https://web.archive.org/web/20170111172309/https://scholarlyoa.com/individual-journals/

3. Least publishable units. http://en.wikipedia.org/wiki/Least_publishable_unit

4. The Northwestern University Collaborative Learning and Integrated Mentoring in the Biosciences (CLIMB) website provides useful information in a series of short webinars. http://www.northwestern.edu/climb/resources/written-communication/index.html

5. Committee on Publication Ethics (COPE). http://publicationethics.org/ This site includes many case studies of real problems related to responsible authorship.

6. International Committee of Medical Journal Editors. www.icmje.org. An international group of medical editors provides guidance on authorship, ethical writing and reviewing and much more.

7. The Elements of Style by William Strunk, Jr. and E. B. White, 4th edition, 1999 Longman. Every writer should have this book.

8. Essential of Writing Biomedical Research Papers 2nd ed Mimi Zeiger. This book covers every detail of how to write a paper from the choice of words, construction of sentences and paragraphs, and packaging of the paper.

Chapter 9
Writing a paper – how to respond to reviewers

Every paper you submit will be rejected

Dear Dr. X, I regret to inform you that we are unable to accept your paper for publication.... You will become familiar with this email; every paper you submit is likely to be rejected, at least initially. What matters most are the sentences that follow the initial statement of rejection and how you respond.

Not every rejection is a rejection

Many rejection letters are, in fact, qualified endorsements of your paper and contain an invitation for you to submit a revised manuscript. These invitations are seldom enthusiastic because the editor does not want to give you the expectation that your revision will be accepted. Nevertheless, most journals (other than very high-impact journals) accept the majority of revised manuscripts. Therefore, no matter how unenthusiastic the letter seems, if a journal offers you the opportunity to revise and resubmit, even as a "*de novo*" submission, do so. A real letter of rejection is unambiguously final (e.g., "will not be considered further" or "good luck with publishing your excellent work in another journal").

If invited, almost always resubmit

Once you have your foot in the door, keep knocking until it opens or you are locked out. Invitations to resubmit from some journals, particularly high-impact journals, are so funereal in tone that the novice is tempted to weep and move on. That is a mistake. A gloomy letter from a high-impact journal dangling the possibility of resubmitting is actually a love letter (mentor Alastair Wood). Inexperienced investigators may crumble at the wording of such a rejection letter and resolve to move on another journal until the mentor looks at the letter and shocks the mentee by saying, "They like your paper, I think it has a good chance if we fix it."

Besides, what have you got to lose? If you send the paper to a different, lower-ranked journal there is no guarantee the reviews will be any kinder, or that it will be accepted. In fact, lower ranked journals often give you tougher reviews. There are a few situations when it is wise not to revise and resubmit. One is if a reviewer <u>and</u> the editor request additional experiments that you are unwilling to do and cannot argue are unnecessary. But, if only one reviewer requests additional experiments that you cannot do, you should revise and resubmit and carefully explain to the editor why you elected not to do the experiments.

If rejected, almost always take your kicks and move on

If a journal unequivocally rejects your paper, it is almost always wise to accept the decision and move on. Do not fire off angry emails to the editor. You can appeal a rejection, but only if a reviewer made a fundamental error. Disagreements about the worth of a paper are not a basis for appeal, nor are several small reviewer errors. Sometimes the reviews seem much more positive than the editorial rejection letter; this is not grounds for appeal. An editor often rejects a paper because of its priority for the journal. Unless a reviewer says your paper is invalid, and this opinion is incorrect, you don't have strong grounds for appeal.

How to appeal a decision

If you decide to appeal a decision, you can email the editor and explain why an appeal is justified and provide information (including new studies if you have them) that rebuts the reviewer's position. A letter of appeal or rebuttal should be polite and factual with the goal of convincing the editor that your paper is worth another look and that you have a constructive rather than an inflammatory response to criticism. Faced with a letter of appeal, the editor has several options: 1) stand by the decision to reject and explain that the decision was based on priority; 2) send the paper to additional reviewers (often members of the editorial board); 3) ask you to respond to the reviewers and resubmit.

Another way to lodge an appeal is to resubmit the paper with a complete response to reviewers, just as you would have done if you had been asked to revise and resubmit and to include a letter of appeal to the editor.

Q. How do you revise and resubmit? A. With grace

The point of submitting a revision is to get the paper published; it is not to prove the reviewer wrong or to complain about the review process. As someone once reminded me, "Our aim is to get the paper accepted, not to get into a pissing match with the reviewer." Revising a manuscript is an exercise in diplomacy and negotiation. There are 4 keys to a successful revision.

1) Don't whine, bite, or grovel.
2) Throw the reviewers bones (usually).
3) Show you did what they asked.
4) Proofread.

1) Don't whine, bite, or grovel: The tone of your response should be polite, tactful, responsive, and professional. Whining (complaining and then grudgingly doing something) is counterproductive. For example, as a reviewer, how would you feel about the following response? *Reviewer 1 has not read our manuscript carefully enough. There are many instances where the reviewer is incorrect or asks for information that is unnecessary or already present. On page 4 we clearly explained that we used geometric means. Nevertheless, despite our reservations, we have made the changes requested.* Similarly, being confrontational and non-responsive (biting) is unlikely to make the reviewer an advocate for your paper.

Groveling is the other side of the coin: *We thank the esteemed reviewer for these remarkable insights that we totally missed. These outstanding suggestions illustrate the reviewer's extraordinary expertise in the area and will transform the paper.* Occasionally a reviewer does provide a remarkable new insight, and a polite thank you is appropriate, but don't fawn.

2) Throw the reviewers bones (usually): The most responsive approach to a revision is to do what the reviewers ask, and unless there are good reasons not to do so, this is my usual approach. If you cannot do what reviewers ask, at least try to throw them a bone: *Reviewers asked for information about blood pressure levels; we do not have that information, but we have now included information about how many subjects were receiving anti-hypertensive therapy.*

Sometimes reviewers will ask you to repeat analyses in a way that is inferior to your current approach. You can either 1) fight the point, crush the reviewer, and hope to win; or 2) do the analysis requested, show the reviewer the result in your response, and diplomatically mention that you have not changed the approach in the paper because your approach is sound.

Sometimes, a reviewer will ask you to delete a figure or table. If you want to keep it, one way to do so and remain responsive is as follows: *We prefer to keep Figure 2 because it illustrates xyz; however, if the editor believes it would improve the paper, we will move it to an on-line supplement.*

If a reviewer asks you to do something that is wrong, you should not do it. Diplomatically explain why your approach is correct and the reviewer's less ideal (without using words such as stupid, poor, wrong, incorrect, ill-informed, ill-conceived, or foolish). Picking a fight with the reviewer is counterproductive.

3) Pat the dog – show the reviewers you did what they asked: Respond to reviewers succinctly and point by point. Do not omit some of their points. Tell them how you have changed the manuscript. It is helpful to include each reviewer's comments and then your response in a different font or type. Usually, reviewers number their comments – if not, do so yourself. The examples that follow illustrate different approaches. The "Bad Responses" may be correct, but they will not make the reviewer your advocate.

Examples of responses to reviewers

Reviewer 1

1. I suggest you construct composite dose-response curves for both groups.

Good Response: Constructing averaged dose-response curves for groups can be problematic because of the large interindividual variability of responses. (This is a tactful way of saying that our initial approach was more correct, but notice in the next sentence that we try to accommodate the request and keep our initial approach.) We have constructed averaged dose-response curves for the groups. The responses estimated from the averaged group were remarkably similar to those derived from individual dose-response graphs (Table 1), thus we have not added this information to the manuscript. (You have thrown the reviewer a bone by doing what was asked, and although you decided not to include that information in the paper, you have provided it to the reviewer.)

Bad Response (whining and biting): The reviewer asks us to combine the dose-response curves for individuals in the two groups. This is not the right way to analyze the data because of the large variability between individuals. Experts would support our approach, and what the reviewer suggests would not be sanctioned. Despite the flawed approach and our reservations, we did nevertheless construct the figure and it shows exactly what we found with our original correct analysis.

2. Please provide a more detailed analysis regarding factors influencing response. For example, did blood pressure and body mass index affect the response?

Good Response: As suggested, we have performed analyses with additional covariates. In a model that included age, sex, body mass index, and blood pressure none of the covariates was significantly associated with response and the outcome was not changed. (The preceding sentence accommodates the reviewer and tactfully makes the point that the initial approach was sound.)

Bad Response (biting): The reviewer asks us to add additional covariates to the model without presenting any reasonable explanation to justify the requested covariates. Statistical rigor dictates that because these covariates were not specified *a priori*, we should not perform the analysis.

3. The first sentence of the discussion should be toned down. There is very large overlap in response between the two groups although the mean response is different.

> **Good Response**: As suggested, we have rephrased the beginning of the Discussion as follows: "The major finding of this study is that on average women appear more…

> **Bad Response (biting)**: Our statement was true and therefore we have not changed it.

4. Indicate what ECG and BMI stand for.

> **Good Response:** Done.

> **Bad Response (groveling):** We thank the diligent reviewer for drawing our attention to this inadvertent omission that occurred despite our best efforts. We greatly appreciate the guidance and expertise of the reviewer and have made every effort to improve the manuscript according to excellent suggestions such as these.

4) Proofread: When I revise a manuscript, I first finish the response to reviewers (this takes several drafts) and then make changes to the manuscript. In this way I can cut and paste sentences from the response to reviewers directly into the revised manuscript. On the other hand, some of my colleagues do it the opposite way. They first revise the paper and then cut and paste from the revised paper into the letter. Whichever way works best for you, show your changes because most journals ask to see a version of the manuscript that shows them. Use "track changes" or highlighting to do this.

A revision is an opportunity to take a fresh look at the paper – if you find errors you must correct them. If the error is serious; for example, a change in a P-value that alters a conclusion, you must briefly tell the editor what happened. Don't try to sneak important changes into the paper without mentioning them. You will look both sloppy and sneaky. Some authors are lazy; they believe that because the paper is almost accepted it is not worth spending more effort on it. A sloppy revision with errors and typos reflects poorly on you and your work (and may be rejected). Make sure all co-authors, particularly the senior author, contribute to the response to reviewers and see and approve the final version.

What happens to your revised submission?

The editor who examines your response to the reviewers and the revised paper has several options: 1) if the changes were minor and you show you have addressed them, the editor might accept the paper without additional external review; 2) if the changes were modest but in areas outside the editor's expertise (e.g., statistics), the editor might send your revision back to one or more of the reviewers for comment; 3) if the changes were moderate or large (code for this in the original editor's letter is "major revision required" or "*de novo* resubmission"), the editor will likely send the paper back to the reviewers; 4) if your paper is controversial or reviewers had fundamental disagreements, the editor might send your revision to not only the original reviewers but also new reviewers. You can see that the review process for a revised manuscript can take several weeks.

Should you call the editor about a revision?

It is seldom necessary to call an editor. Editors often view a request for a telephone call as an attempt to curry favor. It is usually better to communicate by email. If you believe a reviewer is being unfair or unreasonable and you have reached an impasse, you can diplomatically inform the editor in your cover letter – with clear reasons for your concerns. This is seldom necessary. Except for rare situations, it is not helpful to criticize a reviewer.

When I was an editor, authors would call me for many other reasons: My competitor has a paper like this under review and I need to get this published as soon as possible. I need to be able to say that my paper is accepted in order to graduate. When will you make a decision? Is John Smith one of the reviewers? Such calls are not in your best interests.

What if you are asked to submit a second revision (R2)?

If a journal asks you to submit a second revision you should do so and approach it just like a first revision. There are several possible reasons for a second request. For example, 1) there may be minor editorial details that need to be fixed before final acceptance (e.g., formatting of references, word count of abstract) – you can fix these easily; or 2) you have not answered all the reviewers' concerns adequately. Pay great attention to what the reviewers ask and be responsive. Unfortunately, some editors lack courage and require every reviewer to sign off on every point, and some reviewers lack the wisdom to see that there is often more than one acceptable approach. A dogmatic, unreasonable reviewer and a weak editor are a difficult combination. You will need tact, diplomacy, and reason to prevail. Remember, the further your paper proceeds, the more likely it is that the journal will accept it. In other words, a request for a second revision is a good sign.

What happens after your paper is accepted?

Great joy, a journal accepts your paper. What next? Generally, all you have to do is wait for the page proofs and pay the page charges. When the proofs arrive, review them obsessively. It is your last chance to correct errors. It is surprising how many errors occur in the proofs despite the process requiring only the transformation of one electronic document into another. Check every number in the manuscript and pay particular attention to the Tables. Subtle changes in spacing in the Tables can render the information nonsense, or worse, misleading. Editors ask you to return proofs within 48 hours. If you need a few more days, ask. It is better to be correct than quick. In the proof stage, you should only correct errors. This is not the time to rephrase and rewrite. However, if a key paper (e.g., someone did exactly the same study) has been published between when you submitted the paper and received the proofs, you can ask the editor if you can add a few lines to your paper and reference the new paper. The journal will sometimes publish this information as a "note added in proof" at the end of your paper.

Reprints?

Journals will ask if you want to order reprints (for a fee, of course). Reprints are exact replicas of the article and are most often bought by drug companies who want to hand them out. In the old days, academic authors would get requests for reprints from authors in countries or institutions without access to that particular journal. These days, electronic communication has rendered reprints obsolete for most noncommercial authors. Save your money.

Pay for on-line early?

Some journals also offer you the opportunity to pay a fee so that your article is available online immediately to any reader for free. I don't see much point in paying for this service. Most of your colleagues will have immediate online access through academic library subscriptions. Also, if your work was supported by NIH, the paper will be available online for free through PubMed Central (see below) no later than 12 months after publication.

If the paper has NIH funding sources it must be lodged in PubMed Central

If your paper is supported by any NIH funds (even partial support), you are legally responsible for lodging it in PubMed Central. Note, PubMed Central is not the same as PubMed. PubMed is the online site where you can perform literature searches and access abstracts and some full text papers. PubMed Central is an online, full-text repository of papers open to all readers for free. After your paper is lodged in PubMed Central, the full article will be available for general viewing 6 to 12 months later, depending on the policy of the journal in which you published. If you acknowledge NIH funding, many journals lodge your paper in PubMed Central automatically; but, many do not. It can be hard to figure out what an individual journal's policy about lodging papers is; even worse, some say they lodge the papers but then they don't. If the journal does not lodge the paper, one of the authors must do so. Instructions are available (1,2); the process is complicated and can lead to a flurry of emails. Once you have completed the lodging process, your paper will be given a temporary NIHMS number and then a final PubMed Central ID number (PMCID). The PMCID is different from the PubMed ID (PMID).

PMCID numbers are important: There are good reasons (in addition to the legal requirements and good citizenship) to make sure you lodge all your NIH-funded papers on PubMed Central and obtain a PMCID number for each. One reason is that NIH will not release your next year's funding for a grant if you list a paper on your progress report that does not have an NIHMS or PMCID number.

Summary

1. If offered the opportunity to resubmit, do so.

2. Don't whine, grovel, or bite.

3. Respond point by point.

4. Keep your responses brief but say how you have changed the manuscript.

5. Be constructive and diplomatic; avoid fighting words.

6. Pay attention to detail.

7. Lodge work supported by NIH in PubMed Central.

Resources

1. About PubMed Central. http://publicaccess.nih.gov/FAQ.htm

2. Instructions for submitting to PubMed Central.
   http://publicaccess.nih.gov/submit_process.htm

Chapter 10

How to review a paper

THE FLIP SIDE OF WRITING AND REVISING PAPERS is reviewing the work of others. At some stage in your career the following email will arrive: *Dear Dr. X, I would be grateful if you could review a paper submitted for publication....* This email will become familiar, but it may cause you anxiety the first few times it arrives. Most of us are never taught to review papers, and we learn how to do it from the way others reviewed our papers. No one taught me that a reviewer has substantial responsibilities and that you should consider these before you agree to review a paper. A reviewer has the following responsibilities: 1) expertise in the area; 2) no conflict of interest; 3) to maintain confidentiality; 4) to do the review and do it in good time; and 5) to be fair and constructive.

Responsibility 1. Expertise in the area

You must have expertise in the area: It may seem obvious, but you should only review papers that fall within your area of expertise. Sometimes you will get invitations to review papers on topics that you know very little about. This usually happens because you were a co-author on a paper outside your usual area of interest and the editor has run a PubMed search for potential reviewers and come up with your email address. For example, say your area of research is inflammation and you collaborated with someone in a study about depression. You measured inflammatory markers in depressed patients and were a co-author on the paper. You now get invitations to review papers on depression, an area in which you have no expertise.

You do not need expertise in every area of the paper: You do not need to be expert in every area of the paper, but you do need to make your position clear to the editor before you accept the review. For example, if a journal asked you to review a paper about inflammation and clinical subsets of depression, you would need to tell the editor that your area of expertise is inflammation not depression. The editor can then decide whether or not you should proceed with the review.

Responsibility 2. No conflict of interest

Conflict of interest – friends, family, and money: You should not review a paper if you have a significant conflict of interest (Chapter 27). Usually this is obvious. (I've received requests to review a manuscript on which I was a co-author – a large conflict of interest.) You should not review papers if any of the co-authors are colleagues, friends, former trainees, family, from your institution, or collaborators. Also, you should not review a paper if you have potential financial conflicts of interest. Here are some obvious examples: you or your spouse own stock in a company that is submitting a paper about one of its products, or you consult for a company whose product is studied. Sometimes, the line of demarcation is not obvious. If you are uncertain, ask the editor. For example, a journal asks you to review a paper and you notice that you once published a paper with one of the authors. That paper was a consensus document and included many co-authors. You have no other relationship with the author. Technically, the author is a collaborator because you have published together. In reality, most editors would not regard this as a significant conflict of interest. You should not review a paper if you have previously reviewed it for another journal.

Conflict of interest – I know the world is flat: You should not review a paper if you have a scientific conflict of interest. Working in the same scientific area is not necessarily a conflict of interest. In fact, if you are asked to review a paper, it is likely that you work in the same area. A conflict arises if there are polarized views in an area and you hold strong, inflexible opinions that might be thought to affect your ability to provide an unbiased review.

Conflict of interest – doing the same study: You also face a conflict of interest when a paper describes experiments virtually identical to ones you are performing. It is tempting to review the paper to see what they did and what they found. The problem is that you could be seen as having used this information to alter your own experiments. You could also be seen as having a bias to slow the review process and accelerate your own experiments. In other words, people might speculate that you gamed the review process by being a slow and demanding reviewer in order to publish your own findings first. If you ask, many scientists believe they have been on the receiving end of such behavior. As a reviewer, it is prudent to avoid this situation.

Conflict of interest – you stole my idea: What if you are working on a scientific problem that is related to the paper you are asked to review and your studies could be thought to have flowed from information in the paper? My advice is to contact the editor, specify what you are doing, and ask if you should be a reviewer. This serves two purposes. First, it brings the potential scientific conflict of interest into the open. Second, it inoculates you against possible future aspersions from the authors that, "You must have reviewed our paper because you stole the idea to do the next set of experiments."

Responsibility 3. Maintain confidentiality

Confidential means confidential: Manuscript reviews are confidential. That means you cannot share the manuscript or any information about it. If you want to show the manuscript to anyone (e.g., your friendly statistician in the office next door to ask about the data analysis), you need to ask the editor for permission. Because the review process is confidential, you cannot under any circumstances contact the authors. If key information is missing from the paper, contact the editor not the authors. You should destroy copies of the manuscript after you have heard the final decision about the paper.

Here are some examples of breaches of confidentiality that I know about.

- A reviewer decided to use a manuscript review as a teaching opportunity and circulated the manuscript to a group of fellows and they discussed the paper and reviewed it together.

- A reviewer sent the paper to others who were doing similar work because "they would find it interesting."

- A reviewer took figures from the paper under review and included them in a talk he was giving (and in the talk said he was reviewing this really interesting paper).

- A reviewer contacted the authors because a figure was illegible.

- A reviewer posted a copy of the unpublished paper on his personal website.

Responsibility 4. Do the review, do it well, and do it in good time

Do it: Once you have agreed to do a review you are responsible for doing it; other than death or serious illness there are almost no acceptable excuses. You cannot, after the fact, change your mind or decide that you are too busy. The editor will usually seek two or three reviewers for a paper. If you renege at the last minute, the editor has to find a new reviewer and that delays the process and is unfair on the authors and the editor.

Do it well: You should do a thorough and thoughtful review. If you skim the paper and dash off a few comments you will move it off your desk but you abrogate your responsibility. If you do a good review you help the editors, the authors, and the world of science. All serious scientists are concerned about low quality, open-access, fee-for-publication journals that have proliferated and publish papers after minimal or poor quality reviews. For example, John Bohannon of *Science* magazine tested the system and submitted a badly flawed paper to 304 online journals. More than half the journals accepted the paper (1).

Do it in good time: The editor sets a deadline for reviews, usually 2-4 weeks. From a time-management perspective, the review will consume a fixed unit of time whether you do it today or in three weeks time. It takes me approximately 2-4 hours to review a paper. Plan to do the review well before the deadline and move it off your desk. Editors get exasperated when they have to chase down recalcitrant reviewers who have not responded to automated email reminders.

Authors are frustrated when they follow the progress of a manuscript on-line and see that it is still "out for review" 8 weeks after they submitted it. Editors and authors appreciate prompt, thoughtful reviews. The only potential downside of doing reviews within a couple of days is that the same journal may ask you to do more reviews.

Responsibility 5. Be fair and constructive

If you cannot be fair and constructive, you should not do the review.

Why should you review papers?

With all these responsibilities, you might wonder why anyone agrees to review a paper. We review for several reasons, some altruistic, and some selfish. The scientific world turns on our altruistic collaborative efforts. We review papers and try to do it well because we know that the quality of scientific information is important. We hope that just as we review the papers of others, others will review ours. In other words, scientific good citizenship is an important reason to review papers. We also review papers because we learn something. You almost always only review papers in an area that you are particularly interested in. If you review a paper, you get access to the latest ideas in your field before they are published.

Should you say yes?

When the invitation arrives, your first decision is how to respond. If you meet the responsibilities of a reviewer and have time to do the review, you should usually say yes. Unless I have a good reason not to do so, I agree to review for a journal that I want to publish in. Also, you should agree to review a paper if a high-impact journal invites you, or if an editor you know personally asks. If you particularly want to review a paper, accept the invitation quickly. Editors often invite several reviewers and then the automated system accepts the first 2 or 3 that agree (first-come-first-served).

Should you say no or ignore it?

You should turn down a request to review if you are conflicted or too busy. You will also receive requests to review for journals that are low-quality, commercial ventures, sometimes called predatory journals (Chapter 8). I usually ignore these requests because I don't want them to add me to their email lists.

How many reviews should you do?

If you review well and efficiently, an editor might ask you to review again. You may get more requests to review than you can handle and need to limit the number you accept. Doing reviews strengthens your portfolio for promotion (Chapter 20) and is part of being a good scientific citizen but it also takes time away from your own research. I usually review only one paper at a time and not more than one (occasionally two) a month. If I am reviewing grants, I don't undertake manuscript reviews at the same time. These are my preferences – you will develop your own. A journal that asks you to review more than approximately four articles a year may be taking advantage of your goodwill. Perhaps that particular journal should consider you for a position on the editorial board if your opinion is that important. Do not accept invitations to join the editorial boards of questionable journals.

How to review the paper

Search and read the paper: When you start your review the first thing to do is run a PubMed search to make sure this is not a duplicate publication, and to scan recent publications in the area. Read the paper with an open mind and avoid a rush to judgment. I print the paper and scribble notes to myself. Often questions that I asked myself early in the paper are clarified later. Then I put the paper aside for a day or two, think about it, and then re-read it before writing the review.

As you read the paper, ask yourself why the authors did the study, how they did it, and how they interpreted what they found. Editors select articles to publish based on their novelty, importance, interest, and validity. So, also ask yourself the following questions. What is the new information? Is the finding potentially important? Is the question interesting? Based on the approach, how likely is it that the findings are true?

Write your review in a bland tone: Write your review in numbered points using a bland, factual tone that is free of emotion, insult, and praise. Make your points tactfully without causing offence (Table). If you gush about a paper, for example: *The authors are to be congratulated on performing this extremely important and flawless study*, you make it difficult for an editor to reject the paper without setting off a firestorm of correspondence from the aggrieved authors.

Keep the tone bland	
NO	**YES**
Absolute rubbish	Has limited appeal
Egregious error	Authors may be mistaken
Written by a 7-year old	English would benefit from greater attention
The authors are naïve	The authors appear not to have considered
Fatally flawed	A major concern that may not be able to be remedied
This outstanding paper will revolutionize care and should be published	The work is interesting and potentially important

Comments for the editor – new, important, interesting, valid, suitable: Most journals ask you to separate your review into two sections, one for the editor and the other for the authors. When I started reviewing, I thought the two sections existed for logistic convenience and I copied the same review into both sections. In fact, the editor also reads your comments to the authors. Your comments to the editor and those to the authors serve different purposes. The editor may not know your scientific area, and benefits from frank comments about the novelty, importance, and validity of the paper. Also, editors want to know how interesting the paper is and if it is suitable for a particular journal. Your comments to the editor are almost never shared with the authors, and you can be more direct here than in your comments to authors. Nevertheless, keep a professional, judicial tone.

Comments for the editor – red flags: If you believe a paper is invalid because it has flawed methods, you must say so in your comments to the editor. Also, if there are red flags about ethics, libel, plagiarism, or manipulation or fabrication of data, you should tell the editor what is worrying you. You don't need to accuse the authors of anything, but if you diplomatically draw the editor's attention to an area that worries you, the responsibility is on the editor to evaluate it. On the other hand, you should be responsible and report facts – raising questions because of a gut feeling is unfair.

Comments for the authors: The comments for the authors focus on the details of how they performed, interpreted, and presented the study, and do not address whether the paper is suitable for publication or not. I find it easiest to structure the comments to authors under two subheadings. The first, "General Comments," summarizes my thoughts that are relevant to more than one section of the paper. The second, "Specific Comments," focuses on each section in turn (see example review below). Your comments, even if they are critical, should be constructive and draw attention to errors, omissions, lack of clarity, bias, alternative ways of interpreting the data, statistical and methodological weaknesses, and the clarity of the Tables and Figures. You should comment on the writing and grammar if they detract from the paper. If a few typos have escaped the authors' attention, point them out; however, it is not your job to fix the English and edit the paper line by line. Number your comments. Don't toot your own horn (and lose your anonymity) by asking the authors to cite your papers unless they have missed a reference that is absolutely critical.

An example of a review

Comments for editor

This paper represents a lot of work but is largely confirmatory. The importance of the work, as currently formatted, is modest. However, there is little information about this topic and the question is interesting to oncologists. The writing and grammar need extensive copyediting. Apart from the multiple statistical tests, the Methods seem sound but there are so many statistical comparisons that the paper is confusing. The authors do not communicate the major finding – the apparent decrease in platelet numbers over time with drug X – convincingly. The authors do not cite and discuss the Smith paper I have referred them to. Smith did a very similar study with opposite findings. The subject of the paper is suitable for the journal. I think they can address all the issues raised; therefore, whether you accept or reject the paper depends on your assessment of its priority for the journal and how the paper is revised.

Comments for authors

General Comments

The authors performed a randomized controlled study comparing platelet responses over time when patients were exposed to drug X or drug Y. They suggest that X causes a delayed decrease in platelet count between days 72 and 96.

1. It would be helpful if the authors explained to the reader what is novel and what is confirmatory and cite previous papers that examined the platelet response to X and Y.
2. I suggest they cite and discuss the paper by Smith AB et al *J Res Examples* 2016;24:287-295. Specifically, Smith (with a similar design) did not find the decrease over time in platelet counts.
3. There are many grammatical errors; the writing would benefit from careful copyediting.

Specific Comments

1. Abstract: Please make clear in the abstract what was done. Please indicate if the time to response (12 vs. 9 days) is median or mean, and please provide IQR or SD (both in the abstract and the paper).
2. Introduction: line 3 – reads as though the metabolite of X was studied whereas I think X was studied. Need to cite other papers that have looked at the time effect.
3. Methods: Many statistical tests were performed – should acknowledge this and the problems it may cause. There is no sample size justification.
4. Results: The apparent decrease in platelet count over time in those receiving X between days 72 and day 96 is not convincing. Please provide actual numbers (mean with SD or median with IQR).
5. Discussion: Discuss the Smith paper I mentioned.
6. Figures: There are a lot of Figures, many are not particularly helpful. I suggest you delete some of them. In Figure 1 it would be helpful to also show doses of X and Y.
7. There are too many references (93) for a paper in this journal. I suggest the authors reduce them by at least 50 percent.

Do you wish to see the revision?

There is often a box on the reviewer's form that asks you to indicate whether you wish to see the revision. I am not sure why editors ask this question; an editor should make this decision based on how complex the revision is. I usually check the "No" box, but many revised papers arrive for a second review anyway. I know many reviewers who always check the "Yes" box, because they feel responsible for making sure the authors actually do what they need to do.

Do you think the paper warrants an editorial?

There is also sometimes a box that asks if you think the paper warrants an editorial. Give your honest opinion, but if you check "Yes," the editor might ask you to write the editorial or suggest an editorialist.

Accept? Reject? Revise?

There is usually a question that asks if you recommend the editor accept, reject, or reconsider after minor or major revision. I find this question difficult to answer because I don't know the priorities of the journal. If you check the "reconsider after revision" box, you are saying that if the authors deal with all the questions you raised, the paper should be accepted.

What happens after your review is submitted

After all the reviewers submit their reviews, the editor makes a decision. Generally, journals send each reviewer a copy of the editor's decision and the other reviewers' comments. You will find it interesting and educational to read what the other reviewers thought about the paper. Once the review process is over, you must destroy your copy of the paper. You should also update the list of journals you have reviewed for on your CV (Chapter 21).

Summary

Don't do this:	**Do this:**
Renege on reviews or do them late.	Do reviews on time.
Share papers you are asked to review.	Maintain confidentiality
Make sarcastic, personal, or derogatory comments to the authors.	Use tact, diplomacy, and euphemisms.
Play God and expect authors to do everything you suggest.	Be reasonable.
Praise effusively so that it is difficult for the editor to reject the paper.	Keep your tone bland.
Shoot from the hip.	Do a thoughtful review.

Resources

1. Bohannon J. Who's afraid of peer review? Science 2013;342:60-5.

2. Hoppin FG. How I review an original scientific article. Am J Resp Crit Care Med 2002;166:1019-23.

3. Reidenberg JW. Improving peer review: A guide for reviewers of biomedical research. Clin Pharmacol Ther 2002;72:469-73.

Chapter 11
Writing a grant – which one and when?

When do I apply for a grant?

You apply early and often. To become an independent scientist, you will have to be a successful grant writer, and this takes a lot of practice. Apply for grants early in your career and keep applying for them as you advance. It takes approximately 12 months from the time you submit a grant to when funding begins (if you are successful). Therefore, you must apply for grants well ahead of when you need support. Most successful scientists submit at least one or two grants a year. People often paint a gloomy picture of grant writing, and it is true that most grant applications are not funded, but it is also true that the only way to guarantee you won't be funded is not to apply. Grant-writing is a bit like baseball – even the best players strike out a lot but it does not affect their confidence or effort. Or, as one of my mentors said, "If you throw a lot of stuff at the wall, some will stick."

Is there a grant that might support me?

Early-career scientists usually apply for one of two types of grants: career development or research grants. Career development grants get you to your next academic stepping stone and require strong science and an outstanding mentor, environment, and training plan. Different career grants are targeted at different levels; for example, some F and T grants are predoctoral and others postdoctoral and most K-grants facilitate transition from postdoctoral fellow to independent researcher. In addition to NIH, many societies have grants that support career development. However, once you have benefited from a career development grant at a particular career level, you cannot go back to a lower level, nor can you apply for another grant at the same level. Also, you cannot hold two career development grants concurrently. Research grants, on the other hand, are focused on the research project rather than on your career potential, and you may hold several concurrently, provided their scope of work is different. Many funding sources support career development and research grants but three predominate: 1) private and charitable organizations, 2) the Veteran's Administration (VA) and the Department of Defense (DOD), and 3) the National Institutes of Health (NIH).

Private and charitable organizations

Many specialty associations (e.g., American Heart Association) and other nonprofit and charitable organizations (e.g., Lupus Research Alliance, Thrasher Research Fund) offer a range of grants, many aimed at early-career investigators. There are too many potential funding sources to list; explore the websites listed in the Resources section and they will direct you to non-NIH funding. Don't categorize your work too narrowly. For example, even if you are working on diabetes, the American Heart Association might fund your work in obesity and diabetes because these conditions affect cardiovascular health.

Veterans Administration (VA) and Department of Defense (DOD)

You do not have to be a DOD employee to apply for research funding (although it helps). However, to apply for a VA Career Development Award (CDA) you must be nominated by a VA facility and have a VA mentor. If your usual mentor is not on VA staff, you can have a co-mentoring arrangement that includes a VA mentor. Sometimes, the VA mentor is a figurehead for the purpose of the grant and the regular mentor does most of the mentoring. CDAs from the VA are more attractive than NIH K-awards – they provide more salary and research support. VA research grants (equivalent to an RO1) are called Merit awards. If you are a clinician and want to apply for a Merit award, you will need to contact the Director of Research or Chief of Staff at your local VA Medical Center because you must have a VA appointment that pays for at least 5/8ths of your effort. I think it is easier to get a VA grant than an NIH grant; on the other hand, working in the VA is much more bureaucratic, particularly for research that involves humans. DOD grants are usually restricted to particular topics – check the website for details. It may surprise you, but DOD grant opportunities are frequently for diseases that affect mainly women or the elderly.

National Institutes of Health – a complex organization

NIH and its website, processes, instructions, and advice are confusing, constantly changing, and difficult to navigate. NIH has 27 Institutes and Centers (ICs) that focus on different areas. They are often indentified by acronyms; for example, NCI (National Cancer Institute), NHLBI (National Heart, Lung, and Blood Institute), NIGMS (National Institute of General Medical Sciences), and so on. Each IC has a different budget, a different percentile score at which they fund grants (payline), and a different agenda for the type of research and training it promotes. As a result, not all ICs support all types of training grants. Often ICs join to solicit research applications. These solicitations are known as Requests for Applications (RFAs), Request for Proposals (RFPs), and Program Announcement (PAs). A useful online glossary explains NIH terms and acronyms such as these (1).

Different NIH grants

NIH uses an alphanumeric code (e.g., R01, R21, K08, U01) to designate different types of research grants (3). To complicate matters, not all ICs support all types of grants, and if they do support a grant they might have different eligibility criteria. To complicate matters further, since 2018 NIH has designated grants as: clinical trial not allowed; clinical trial optional; and clinical trial required. Remember that NIH's definition of a clinical trial is very different from most people's definition (Chapter 15). Although there are many different types of grants, some are more likely to be relevant to you early in your career; these include T, F, and K grants.

RFAs, RFPs, and PAs

RFAs are often one-time requests for grant applications on a particular topic. The deadline for RFA applications often falls soon after the opportunity is announced, but sometimes RFAs are repeated. RFPs solicit applications for contracts to perform a particular task. NIH usually sets aside a pot of money for RFAs and RFPs to fund successful applications. On the other hand, PAs do not have a pot of earmarked funding, and NIH uses them to build interest in an area. PAs often have several receipt dates and may span several years.

Payline

The payline is the percentile above which a particular IC will fund a grant. If you look at data for NIH paylines you will notice that there is not a rigid cut-off at a certain percentile. In other words, someone with a grant scored in the 14th percentile might not be funded while another person with a score in the 18th percentile is funded. Not fair, you might say. Others say this flexibility allows NIH to structure its research portfolio strategically. PAs and other factors contribute to the flexible funding line.

Finding NIH's solicitations for grants

The NIH puts out a Guide for Grants and Contracts that describes upcoming and current funding opportunities. You should subscribe to receive this weekly email so that you know about upcoming and active RFAs, RFPs, and PAs (collectively known as funding opportunity announcements (FOAs); you can also search for funding opportunities in different disease or scientific areas (2). Remember, you can apply for an unsolicited RO1 on any topic; it is better to stick to your area of expertise than to search for an RFA on some topic tenuously related to your interests and try to cook up an application for that. Recently, some ICs no longer accept unsolicited RO1 applications that involve clinical trials. Since NIH defines clinical trials very broadly (discussed later – but in summary any intervention in a human), the widespread implementation of policies such as this will have serious adverse effects on clinical research.

SROs and POs

The NIH staff members most helpful to you are program officers (POs) and scientific review officers (SROs). They fulfill different roles. POs are responsible for the research direction in the various NIH ICs and will talk to you about the science of your application. For example: is your work interesting to a particular IC; which study section might be suitable; would your proposal be responsive to a particular RFA; how to interpret your summary statement and score. SROs are responsible for overseeing the review of grants. They find reviewers, assign grants for review, and organize the study section. Your usual point of contact is the PO, except for matters related to the review process.

Should you talk to your PO?

People usually advise you to talk to your PO, but opinions differ. Some say it was not helpful because they found it difficult to contact the PO and the advice was vague or even wrong. Others found talking to their PO useful. POs have behind-the-scenes influence on which grants (and therefore which investigators) get funded. Therefore, if a PO is your advocate, you are more likely to get funding. Some (including me) think this is uncomfortably close to political schmoozing, but if this the way the game is played, you should know the rules. To talk to your PO send an email and ask for a time to have a telephone conversation. Your email must provide information about the specific grant application you want to discuss. POs vary a lot in how responsive they are, and if you don't hear back within a week, send another email, and if you still don't hear back, call and leave a message. Never get on the wrong side of a PO – use diplomacy, enthusiasm, and willingness to learn as your tools.

Research training (T and F Grants)

T32 awards (also known as Ruth L. Kirchstein awards): NIH awards T32s to institutions to train researchers in specific areas. Because so many institutions have T32 awards, you will find it virtually impossible to learn about all the open T32 positions. Some institutions advertise their positions, others do not. Often the only way you can find information is to go to department and division websites and search for information about T32 awards. Some T32s are for predoctoral and others for postdoctoral research training. To be a candidate for a T32 you must be a US citizen or permanent resident. To be competitive for a postdoctoral T32 you should have a track record of research, some publications, and a career plan focused on research. Most T32s allow 3 years of support, but many programs limit this to 2 years so they can support more people.

T32 payback rule: NIH has a payback rule for postdoctoral T32s: if you are supported by a T32 for one year and then leave for private practice, you will have to pay back all the money you received (to a maximum of one year's support). If however, after one year on the T32 you move to another university, or to the FDA, or another situation where you are performing research, you will not be required to pay anything back. If you spend two years on the T32, you are in the clear because your second year pays back the first. The goal of the payback rule is to prevent clinical fellows using a year of NIH support as a finishing school for obtaining additional clinical skills and then going into private practice.

F32s: An F32 is virtually identical to a T32 except that NIH grants the F32 to you rather than to your institution. This means that you need to write the grant application and have a position, mentor, and track record in order to be competitive. Some NIH institutes subtract time you have already spent in your mentor's laboratory from your 3 years of possible support on an F32.

Career development awards (K Grants)

You must be a US citizen or permanent resident (green card holder) to be eligible for career development Ks (KO1, K08, K23) other than K99s. Career development Ks generally require that you spend at least 75% of your time doing research or career development activities; they are generally funded for 5 years unless you already have substantial training and the study section thinks you should become independent in a shorter time. Also, K-awards can only support you for a total of 6 years. So if you have received a KL2 or KL12 award (2-3 year awards usually granted by local CTSAs) you may not be eligible for 5 years of support on a K08 or K23. Not all ICs support all types of K-awards, and different institutes have different eligibility rules and different training priorities (4).

There is a sweet spot for career development grants

Career development grants invest in training promising researchers. Therefore, if you are already well trained (overqualified), or if you have not yet shown promise (underqualified), you will be less competitive. It is important to find the sweet spot when you have shown commitment to a research career and had some early success but have not been around for too long with too much success. Reviewers evaluate your career trajectory and its potential according to the number of years of mentored research training you have had and the number and quality of your publications. There is no ideal number for either, but individuals with no publications are underqualified and those with a large number are likely overqualified for K-awards. Many of the K-applications I have reviewed have been from individuals with 6 to 12 publications (some as first author) who have been in research training for 3 to 6 years, but those numbers vary a lot. If you think reviewers might see you as overqualified, you should address the question directly and use your personal narrative section to explain what you are not trained in and how your career development and research plans fill that gap. The median age of K23 and K08 awardees is approximately 37 years.

Mentored research scientist development awards

KO1: For individuals with a clinical or non-clinical doctoral degree (most often PhDs doing basic research).

KO8: For individuals with a clinical doctoral degree (e.g., MD, Pharm D, DO) most often doing basic research but sometimes clinical research that does not involve hands-on patient contact (e.g., epidemiology).

K23: For individuals with a clinical doctoral degree (e.g., MD, Pharm D, DO) doing patient-oriented research.

K99/R00: The "Pathway to Independence Award" is aimed at individuals who are almost ready for independence. It is a hybrid that combines 1-2 years of mentored K-type funding with 3 years of independent R-type funding. It is open to non-U.S. citizens. People who apply for the K99 are more advanced than those applying for other K-awards; they have more publications, have established an independent area of research, and are close to independence.

Research grants

R01: This is the bread-and-butter NIH research grant that is used by all ICs. It usually supports a project for 5 years (if the amount of work justifies it).

R21: This grant is for exploratory research and does not require preliminary data. It is limited to 2 years of funding and the total direct costs in those years cannot exceed $275,000.

R03: This grant is for small limited projects that need support for a short time. For example, it can be used for pilot studies, secondary analysis of existing data, and developing new methods. It is limited to 2 years usually with direct costs of $50,000 per year.

Other grants

Other grants you will come across are multi-investigator P and U-awards. For example, your mentor may be part of a multi-investigator grant supported by a PO1 (Program Project Grant) or a P50 (Specialized Center Grant). Principal investigators for projects on P-grants are almost always established investigators who have had at least one RO1. A UO1 (Research Project Cooperative Agreement) supports special areas of interest and has a lot of hands-on involvement with the IC that funds the grant.

Send your grant to as many places as possible

You can send exactly the same science to a society, the VA, and the NIH. Inefficiently for us, they have different forms and requirements. Thus even sending the same grant to these different places is not a trivial matter, but it does increase your chance of funding 3-fold. One reviewer often determines whether your grant will be funded, so there is a large element of randomness; therefore, the more grants you have in play the greater your chances of success. Of course, if you are lucky and more than one funding source wants to fund your grant, you can only accept one. Also, except under very specific circumstances, you cannot send multiple versions of the same grant to NIH at the same time. One exception is that you can simultaneously submit the identical grant as an R application and also as a project in a multi-investigator P-award.

New Investigators and Early Stage Investigators

NIH definition of New Investigator: A New Investigator is a PI who has not previously been the PI of a substantial NIH independent research award (e.g., an RO1). A person who has been PI of a smaller grant (e.g., an RO3) or was supported by a training grant would qualify (5).

NIH definition of Early Stage Investigator: An Early Stage Investigator (ESI) is a New Investigator who is within 10 years of completing a terminal research degree or completing medical residency (5).

It is good to be an ESI: NIH makes special allowances for applications from New Investigators and ESIs during both peer review and consideration for funding. NIH asks reviewers to expect less preliminary data and to pay less attention to past achievements. Also, NIH ICs have more generous paylines and shift the funding percentile so that the same proportion of new investigator and established investigator applications are funded. An unresolved concern is that for some investigators this turns out to be a mixed blessing – getting the first grant was possible but the next hits a brick wall. NIH is now considering special dispensations for investigators who are within ten years of their first RO1 award.

Summary

1. It is complicated to figure out which grants are suitable for you. Your mentors must guide you and you must look for grants actively.

2. Write grants early and often in your career.

3. The only way to guarantee you will not be funded is to not apply.

4. Subscribe to an email from NIH with updates about funding opportunities.

5. Send the same grant to several places to increase your chance of success.

Resources

1. Glossary of NIH terms and acronyms.
   http://grants.nih.gov/grants/glossary.htm#R24

2. To enroll for a weekly email of NIH funding opportunities.
   http://grants.nih.gov/grants/guide/listserv_dev.htm

3. For information about different types of NIH grants:
   http://grants.nih.gov/grants/funding/funding_program.htm
   http://grants.nih.gov/grants/funding/ac_search_results.htm

4. About K-awards. http://www.niddk.nih.gov/research-funding/process/apply/about-funding-mechanisms/k-awards/Pages/K-Awards.aspx

5. New and early stage investigators.
   https://grants.nih.gov/policy/new_investigators/index.htm#definition

6. To find non-NIH sources of funding explore these sites.
   http://oedb.org/ilibrarian/100_places_to_find_funding_your_research/
   http://pivot.cos.com/funding_main

7. To find out about Department of Defense funding for research.
   http://cdmrp.army.mil/funding/default.shtml

8. For information about US Department of Veterans' Affairs grants.
   http://www.research.va.gov/funding/default.cfm

9. A starting point for all NIH grant-related matters.
   http://grants.nih.gov/grants/oer.htm

10. To search for NIH grants in a particular area.
    http://grants.nih.gov/funding/index.htm

Chapter 12

Writing a grant – the layout and style

Writing the grant is the easiest part

The science of an NIH grant is only 13 pages long: 1 page of aims and 12 pages of science. For a K-application these 12 pages also include your career development plan. Most college students, with the help of caffeine, can knock out a good 13-page paper in a weekend. Unfortunately, good grants do not get funded. Many outstanding grants do not get funded. The smallest margins and some luck separate funded and unfunded grants. It takes a lot of time to write a good grant; it can take me a year or longer. I spend most of this time thinking about what I am going to do and constructing the Specific Aims. Once the ideas and the Specific Aims are solid, you can easily write the rest of the grant. Layout and style are important but cannot compensate for poor Aims.

Layout – don't squeeze the text

The layout of grants is fairly standard. The most popular font is 11 point Arial and the most popular margins are 0.5 inches all around. If you can manage it, bigger margins (e.g., 0.6 inches all around) are kinder to readers. You can use a smaller font in the figure legends and tables – often Arial 9 point. Everyone is tempted to squeeze as much writing as possible into the grant. You can do this by leaving no space between paragraphs, having long, dense paragraphs, using few tables or figures, and playing with line spacing. These strategies will indeed squeeze more text onto your 13 pages of science, but they do your grant a disservice. A reviewer's heart sinks at the sight of page upon page of dense unbroken text. Your grant should be pleasing to the eye.

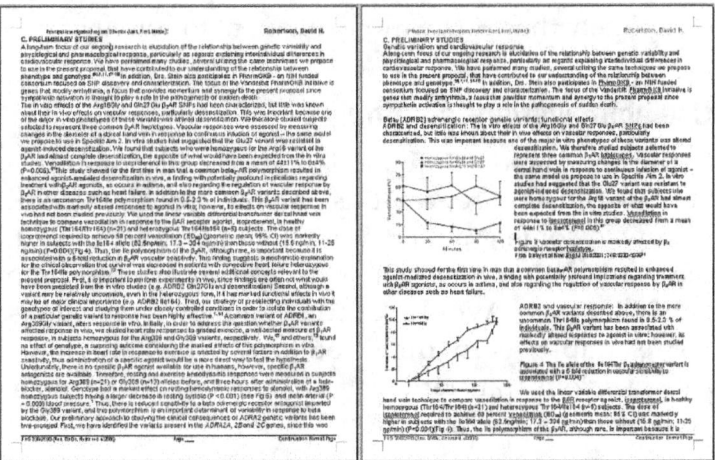

Layout – make it pleasing to the eye

In addition to having some white space, another way you can make a page appealing is to have at least one figure or table per page. Consider the visual effects of the left and right pages – they contain the same information, but the page with figures and some white space is more attractive.

Figures must send a clear message – the legend trumpets the message

Figures in grants are more than scattered decorations. A figure in a grant, just as is the case for figures in a paper (Chapter 7), must send a clear visual message. The message can be simple (e.g., groups A and B look different, or groups C and D do not look different). You have a problem if a reviewer looks at the figure and questions your message. If your message is that two groups are different, then they should indeed look convincingly different. You can make it easy for the reviewer to interpret the figure if the legend summarizes your message. For example, *Patients with metabolic syndrome (Group A) have 3.6-fold higher CRP concentrations than those without (Group B) (P=0.003)* is a much more informative legend for a figure than *CRP concentrations in patients with and without metabolic syndrome.*

Figures must be legible and provide details

It seems obvious, but a figure must be legible to be useful. When you shrink a figure the text can become illegible. Design your figures with large text so that they shrink well. Figures draw attention, and a reviewer will look very critically at what you might regard as a mere illustration. Therefore, figures must have error bars and indicate if these represent SD, SEM, or 95% CI, and the text in the legend must indicate how many experiments or subjects you studied and provide a P value. It is helpful if you can make figures self-standing; in other words, a reviewer who looks at only the figure and its legend should understand completely the information you want to convey.

Use abbreviations sparingly

Limit non-standard abbreviations. Spell out each abbreviation the first time you use it and repeat this in the footnotes to figures and tables. I have reviewed some grants that included a Table of all the abbreviations used and the explanation for each. This approach does help the reviewer, but it uses valuable space. Avoid allocating your own meanings to standard abbreviations. For example, each time you use the abbreviation BMI it will trigger the subconscious translation "body mass index" even if you designated it to mean "bilateral mastoid injections."

Use emphasis sparingly

You can emphasize a handful of key sentences or phrases in the grant to draw a reviewer's attention to particular points. However, it is <u>irritating</u> when you emphasize apparently **random** phrases *or* words by **underlining**, *bolding* or <u>italicizing</u>.

Use bold paragraph headings

Just as is the case with papers (Chapter 8), your paragraphs should be relatively short (approximately eight lines), focused on a single thought, and have a bold heading that identifies that thought – similar to the style of this book. The bold paragraph headings make it easy for the reviewer to find information, follow your argument, and speed read through familiar sections. Unlike this book, in grants I often put the the bold paragraph heading and first line of text on the same line to save space.

Use consistent terminology

You should be consistent in the way you use terminology and units. For example, if you use the terms waist circumference, waist, WC, central adiposity, girth, and truncal obesity to all mean the same thing, you will confuse the reviewer. If you express serum cholesterol as mg/dL in one place and as mmol/L in another, you will confuse everyone.

Avoid hyperbole, cliché and error

Few findings are earth shattering, revolutionary, incredibly important, or unique. Bench-to-bedside is venerable but jaded. State-of-the-art, internationally renowned, children-are-not-small adults, key players, and cutting edge are clichéd. Reviewers have many pet peeves – an important one to avoid is principle investigator. Principle relates to a fundamental belief, <u>p</u>rincipal is the most important. Most of us use the word comprise incorrectly, and if we do use it correctly, the sentence often looks odd. I avoid comprise and use composed of or another substitution. There are many other words that we misuse frequently – spend some time with Strunk & White (1).

Be positive

Replace the following phrases – we plan to, we hope, we will try, we will endeavor, we will attempt – with we will. Avoid the phrases we will thus confirm and we will set out to confirm; they say that your studies are at best confirmatory.

Revise, revise, revise

Small differences separate grants that are funded from those that are not. You can improve your chances by revising your grant for grammar, punctuation, spelling, and clarity. Grants do not sink because of bad grammar, but a reviewer is less likely to become your advocate if your writing is sloppy. Reviewers roll their eyes when they find obvious evidence that you have cut-and-paste a paragraph from another grant and been too lazy or careless to change wording not pertinent to your current application.

Solicit your own reviewers

Ask other people to criticize your grant before you submit it. This is particularly useful at two stages. First, ask reviewers (mentors, senior colleagues) to comment on the Specific Aims page before you write the grant. Listen to their comments. If your Specific Aims are a problem, the rest of the grant is irrelevant. Second, seek reviews when you have finished the grant and it is as good as you can get it.

Internal reviewers are not your copyeditors

Internal reviewers do you a favor by reading your grant – they do not want to read the early versions and correct your spelling and formatting errors. They should focus on key weaknesses. Your mentor will read the grant a few times, but it is not your mentor's job to provide you with Specific Aims, write pieces of the grant, or correct your grammar and spelling. Your mentor and other reviewers contribute most when they identify weak areas that you could strengthen.

Respect your internal reviewers

Be sensitive to your internal reviewers' time. If on Friday you ask for reviews of a grant that you have to submit on Monday, it is disrespectful to the reviewers because it asks them to march to your timetable. Also, the review is irrelevant because there is not enough time for you to make substantive changes no matter what the reviewers say. In this situation, you will often get brief unhelpful reviews, "looks good, best of luck."

Meet your internal reviewers face to face

You will get the most out of internal reviewers if you can get two of them to sit at a table with you for an hour or two and dissect your grant section by section. By doing this you can see where the reviewers agree, where they disagree, and discuss strategies to deal with weaknesses.

Summary

1. Make your application pleasing to the eye.

2. Try to have a figure or table on most pages.

3. Make sure your figures and their legends send the correct message.

4. Make sure your figures can withstand critical questions.

5. Use paragraph headings, short sentences, short paragraphs, and clear language.

6. Eliminate careless errors.

7. Solicit reviews.

Resources

1. The Elements of Style by William Strunk, Jr. and E. B. White, 4 edition 1999 Longman. Every writer should have this book.

2. The Northwestern University Collaborative Learning and Integrated Mentoring in the Biosciences (CLIMB) website provides very useful information in a series of short webinars. http://www.northwestern.edu/climb/resources/written-communication/index.html

3. The Grant Application Writers Workbook. National Institutes of Health Version. Robertson JD, Russell SW and Morrison DC. Grant Writers Seminars and Workshops, LLC (2018). A useful book that covers all components of grant writing and submission.

Chapter 13
Writing a grant – the science

Who are the reviewers and what are they thinking?

The most important principle for writing a fundable grant is for you to think like a reviewer. Reviewers are busy scientists who review grants for different reasons, most often good citizenship. They add these grant reviews to their other work, so they are overworked, overcommitted, and harried speed readers. Even when they start with a positive attitude, they can rapidly become hypercritical curmudgeons. They are often reading grants on the plane, watching a child's soccer match with one eye, or between patients in clinic. You might think that reviewers want to savor every word of your grant. In reality, they are probing for weaknesses to put your application into one of 3 boxes defined by the NIH scoring system (high, medium or low impact) as efficiently as possible

NIH scoring system

<u>High Impact (The perhaps box)</u>
1= Exceptional (exceptionally strong with essentially no weaknesses)
2= Outstanding (extremely strong with negligible weaknesses)
3= Excellent (very strong with only some minor weaknesses)

<u>Medium Impact (The hospital bed)</u>
4= Very Good (strong but with numerous minor weaknesses)
5= Good (strong with at least one moderate weakness)
6= Satisfactory (some strengths but also some moderate weaknesses)

<u>Low Impact (The coffin)</u>
7= Fair (some strengths but at least one major weaknesses)
8= Marginal (a few strengths and a few major weaknesses)
9= Poor (very few strengths and numerous major weaknesses)

How the reviewer puts you in a box

Reviewers read your grant to understand what you want to do and then identify the strengths and weaknesses of your approach. They are like dentists probing with sharp implements – once they have found one or more cavities (say one moderate or several minor weaknesses), their review is over – you will not be funded. Your job is to present a grant that has no weaknesses. To do that you cannot view the grant from your own perspective – a carefully crafted product of months of work by a talented investigator. Instead, you must view it from a reviewer's perspective – an idea that compels the reviewer to fund it.

Answer the reviewer's questions before they are asked

The primary reviewer of your grant will have to sit around a table and explain to other scientists why your grant should score well. Your job is to make it easy for the reviewer to do this. Fortunately, reviewers ask themselves predictable questions and you should write your grant to answer these before they are asked. In fact, the answers to many of the questions should be obvious after reading just the Specific Aims page.

What reviewers ask

As they read, reviewers are constantly asking different versions of the *so what?* question.

- What is the question?
- Why is the question important?
- What is the knowledge gap the study will fill?
- Is it vitally important to fill this knowledge gap?
- Are the proposed studies new?
- If the idea is not new, is there a compelling reason to do the studies?
- Is there a testable hypothesis?
- Is the approach sound (best model, best drug, best analysis, great team)?
- Are there strong preliminary data?
- Are the studies proposed feasible?
- Will the studies elucidate fundamental mechanisms?
- If everything works, what is the deliverable?

The structure of the science section of an NIH grant

The science of an NIH grant is divided into 5 sections: Abstract, Specific Aims, Significance, Innovation, and Approach. Each section is important, but you should pay particular attention to the Abstract and Specific Aims sections because that is all most members of the study section read. Let's discuss the Specific Aims first because this is where you should start when you write a grant.

Specific Aims

The Specific Aims section is only one page, but is the most important part of the grant. This page summarizes what you want to do and why it is important. If the reviewer is not enthusiastic about the questions you are asking after reading this section, your grant is lost. There is no point in writing the rest of the grant until your Specific Aims are watertight. This means that you should get your mentor and other advisors to work with you on your Specific Aims before you launch into writing the rest of the grant. Although we talk a lot about writing a grant, it is more important to think the grant through.

The key components of the Specific Aims page

The Specific Aims section tells a story, often with key arguments in a particular order.

1. Set the big stage for importance. Your opening sentences usually tell the reviewer that the area you are working in is important. *Cardiovascular disease accounts for the majority of deaths in developed nations...*

2. Identify the area you are working in and its importance. *In population studies high HDL concentrations are associated with lower risk of cardiovascular...*

3. Identify the general problem. *However, at least 3 lines of evidence suggest the HDL function may be more important than HDL concentration; 1... 2...3...*

4. Identify the knowledge gap. *Despite the evidence that HDL function is important, we do not understand the mechanism by which HDL is cardioprotective.*

5. Bring in some preliminary data. *Our preliminary findings show... This suggests that HDL may be cardioprotective by...*

6. State the overall question. *Our overall goal is to define the mechanisms whereby HDL is cardioprotective.*

7. State the Specific Aims. *We will define these mechanisms in three Specific Aims. Aim 1 will test the hypothesis that the x function of HDL is cardioprotective by comparing y in patients with and without ischemic heart disease. Aim 2 will test the hypothesis that....*

8. Close with a sentence or two that reinforce importance, novelty, and what the grant will deliver.

Common criticisms of Specific Aims

Reviewers make several recurrent criticisms of Specific Aims and it is worth designing yours so that they are inoculated.

The Aims lack novelty: This criticism means the reviewer believes that many of the answers you seek are already known, or if previous studies are inconclusive, yours will not provide a definitive answer.

The Aims are not compelling: The reviewer finds your story ho-hum; your grant fails the "so-what" test.

The Aims are vague (or lack focus): The reviewer is unclear what you propose to do and how it answers the questions you have posed. Specific Aims must be specific. *We will examine the effects of beetroot on inflammation* is very different from *We will examine the hypothesis that beetroot reduces inflammation measured by the ACR-20 response in patients with rheumatoid arthritis in a randomized, double-blind, placebo-controlled, proof-of-concept study.*

The Aims depend on each other: You must construct your Specific Aims so that the rationale for doing Aim 2 does not depend on Aim 1 succeeding; similarly, Aim 3 cannot depend on the success of Aims 1 or 2. For example, the following Specific Aims are all interdependent: *In Aim 1 we will construct an animal model of x; Aim 2 will define which factors determine y using this model; Aim 3 will examine the factors identified in mice in Aim 2 in a human population.* If Aim 1 does not work, Aims 2 and 3 are doomed. It is a challenge and an art to construct Aims that are related but not interdependent.

The Aims are descriptive and not mechanistic: It is difficult to design mechanistic aims if you are a clinical researcher, but the way you phrase an aim makes a huge difference. For example, contrast *Aim 1 will follow patients with impaired HDL function to determine their course* (100% descriptive) to *Aim 1 will examine the hypothesis that patients with decreased HDL-mediated cholesterol efflux are more likely to develop myocardial infarction in a prospective cohort of 5,000 individuals.* Dan Roden, a very successful grant writer, taught me that certain words and phrases (e.g., define, identify, test an hypothesis, determine mechanisms) are less descriptive than others (e.g., assess, describe, collate, collect, correlate, examine, inspect) and are therefore stronger.

The Aims are overambitious: This criticism means that the reviewer believes you have overestimated your capabilities, and what you propose is not feasible. There is a limit to how much work you can complete in 5 years and how many aims you can address. There is no magic number of aims. Successful grants have had 1, 2, 3, and 4 aims. However, most grants have 3 Specific Aims; this tradition may be due to the idea that if a reviewer hates one aim, then you can omit that aim and resubmit the remaining two as a revised grant. It is reasonable to break aims into subsections; for example, Aim 1a) focuses on the effects of HDL on cholesterol efflux and Aim 1b) focuses on the anti-inflammatory effects of HDL. However, be careful about breaking subsections into further subsections (e.g., Aim 1a (i), 1a (ii) etc.); this can result in very complex Aims that confuse the reviewer.

Abstract

I write the abstract last, after the other components of the science section, because by then my thoughts are clear and easier to summarize. Many of the key components of the Abstract and Specific Aims sections are similar, but the abstract is shorter and often provides a little more detail about how you will do the studies and less detail about the background leading to the proposal. The NIH abstract is a maximum of 30 lines. You must pay attention to the abstract because at the study section meeting (Chapter 18) where reviewers score your grant most people (other than your 3 designated reviewers) only read the Abstract and Specific Aims.

The key components of the abstract

1. Set the stage for importance: why is the disease, problem, or mechanism you address important?

2. Define the knowledge gap.

3. Allude to preliminary results showing that you can fill the knowledge gap (i.e., the rationale for the study).

4. State your overarching hypothesis

5. Describe what you propose to do (Specific Aims) and provide key information about how you will do the studies (e.g., in a knockout mouse, in humans, in a cell line, in a database, using PET scanning, using a novel lithium MRI etc). Most applicants do not cut and paste the exact wording of the actual aims into the abstract (but some do). A more common approach is to paraphrase each aim in a narrative (e.g., In Aim 1 we will examine the hypothesis that the anti-inflammatory effect of HDL are impaired in patients with ischemic heart disease by comparing the ability of their HDL to inhibit cytokine production *ex vivo* with that of controls.

6. Close with a reminder of how the answer to your question will be important.

Significance

Significance is not a literature review: The Significance section used to be called Background and Significance. I think it was renamed because applicants felt a need to review the background world literature, and reviewers grew weary of reading literature reviews.

Your goal for the Significance section is for the reviewer to "buy" your idea, convinced that the topic is very important, that there is a critical knowledge gap, and that you will fill this gap and thus advance science significantly. If you have not hooked the reviewer by the end of the Specific Aims and Significance sections, the rest of the grant does not matter.

The Significance section sells your grant: Your goal in the Significance section is to bring together pieces of information from the literature and from your preliminary studies to weave a compelling story showing that there is an important problem and you can solve it. This means that you have to know the background literature well and use that information for your story. Be careful that you do not present only the evidence that suits you. Reviewers will recognize this and dismiss your story. The key components of the Significance section act together to convince the reviewer: 1) that the area you are working in is critically important; 2) that there is a vitally important problem in this area facing mankind; 3) that there is a critical knowledge gap impeding progress; and 4) that your preliminary data and skills indicate that you can fill the knowledge gap and therefore help solve the problem and save mankind. I have exaggerated to make the point that you have to ask a new and important question in order to have strong Significance section.

Innovation

Generally, the Innovation section is short (a paragraph or two), but writing it is a challenge because most NIH grant applications are not truly innovative. Rather, most grants describe how they will move the field forward, and not how they will revolutionize the field. Innovation is not the same as importance or novelty. Just because your proposed study has never been done before does not mean it is innovative. Innovation is described in the NIH guidelines for reviewers as follows: "1) challenges or shifts the *status quo* in research or clinical practice using novel concepts, methodologies or interventions; 2) uses methodologies that have advantages over existing methodologies; 3) has improvements or new applications of theoretical concepts or interventions, 4) could bring novelty (in approach, methods, concept) to a broad understanding rather than just a narrow field." Try to use some of this exact wording to describe why your grant is innovative.

Approach

"Forms E" and your Approach: In 2018 NIH introduced new requirements for grant applications that include human subjects and NIH-defined clinical trials. These changes require you to provide specific information under a new section, "Human Subjects and Clinical Trials Information" (Chapter 15). There you must provide your inclusion and exclusion criteria, an extensive protocol, details about your sample size/power calculations and planned statistical analysis, and a timeline. In other words, a lot of what you would usually have included in the Approach section is now found in this new human subjects section. NIH asks you not to repeat the same information in different places. No-one is quite sure how to handle this. What most people are doing in the Approach section is to provide a summary of the information that is in the Human Subjects and Clinical Trials Information section and referring the reader to it for additional details.

There are different ways of writing the Approach section. The headings that follow are an example of how you can describe clinical studies.

Preliminary studies: You can include some preliminary findings in the Significance section, but many people prefer to put them in the Approach section. The Preliminary Studies section can fill a page or two and often has two parts: in the first you briefly describe the research team and their individual achievements relevant to the proposed studies, and the in second you describe the findings of studies you have performed that show you can do the proposed studies and that they are worth doing. Some applicants put all their preliminary studies in one section at the beginning of the Approach. Others present relevant preliminary findings at the beginning of each Aim. Both approaches are fine; choose whichever works best. After the Preliminary Studies section, you can describe your approach to each Specific Aim using the headings that follow.

Specific aim and rationale: It is useful to spend a few lines reminding the reviewer about the Specific Aim and its rationale. For example:

> **SPECIFIC AIM 1: Test the hypothesis that skin glycerol concentrations determined by magnetic resonance imaging are higher in patients with a chronic inflammatory renal disease than controls.**
>
> **Rationale:** Several inflammatory renal diseases are characterized by chronic inflammation, vascular dysfunction and hypertension (references). Evidence in animal studies indicates that skin glycerol concentrations may contribute to both inflammation and vascular dysfunction in the setting of chronic inflammatory renal disease. There is no information regarding skin glycerol in human chronic inflammatory renal disease; our preliminary data indicate that glycerol is higher in this setting and mediates tissue damage.

General Approach: Briefly (in a few lines) summarize your overall approach (e.g., a cross-sectional study in 48 patients with stage IV chronic renal failure and 48 controls matched for a, b and c in whom y will be performed and z measured).

Recruitment: Describe where your patients or subjects will come from and how you will recruit them. Reviewers are always concerned whether what you propose is feasible; provide convincing evidence that you can meet your recruitment goals.

Inclusion and Exclusion Criteria: Think about how you will select study subjects; a table listing criteria is often shorter and clearer than text.

Protocol: Explain how you will do the study (e.g., randomization, control of diet, timing of visits, duration and design of the study). Pay attention to details related to the exposure (i.e., intervention), the primary outcome, and confounders.

Methods: Describe the methods you will use to measure outcomes; these include clinical and laboratory measurements. If you have used these methods before, reference your papers to show the reviewer that you know what you are doing. Sometimes you can bring some preliminary data into this section to show that you can do the studies. If you will use the same methods in each Aim, it is easiest to describe the methods in Aim 1 and then refer to that text in later Aims.

Power and sample size: The section on sample size is often a problem. Some grants, particularly those from basic scientists, do not even include sample size calculations, others describe the calculation in such a way that the reviewer is confused and cannot reproduce the calculation. You should base your sample size calculation on the primary outcome and justify the relevance of the size of the difference that you seek to detect. PSPower is a useful free program for calculating power and sample size (1). When I review grants, I often recalculate the sample size estimations, and if I do not have the information to do so, I question what the applicant wrote.

Analysis: Every grant should have a statistician as part of the team, and the statistician should help write the sample size and analysis sections.

Anticipated results: It is important to tell the reviewer what you expect to find, what those findings will mean, and how you will interpret those that are contrary to your expectations.

Limitations, pitfalls and alternative approaches: In this section you show the reviewer that you have thought deeply about the choices you have made. There are always choices among study designs and approaches. You must justify your choices (e.g., why you chose particular cytokines, or measured bleeding and not survival, or chose a crossover design) and discuss the limitations of your approach and how you will deal with problems that may result from your choices. No study can answer every question; rather than have the reviewer point out what you are not doing, point it out yourself and mention these areas as potential future directions. Remember, rather than shoot yourself in the foot, temper potential weaknesses with strengths. For example: *We chose to study individuals aged between 20 and 40 years, and although this may limit the generalizability of our findings, it has the major advantage of limiting intersubject variability.*

Timeline: Every grant must have a timeline; this is usually a single figure at the end of your grant and it illustrates how you expect the aims to progress over the time of the grant. Look at an example in a successful grant.

Rigor, reproducibility and transparency

To promote reproducible science, NIH has required (since 2016) that applicants specifically address scientific rigor and transparency. You must address the 4 components of rigor that NIH has identified.

1. **The scientific premise:** NIH asks you to consider the relevant positive and negative studies that inform your hypothesis and give weight to their scientific rigor. This is naturally part of the Significance section.

2. **Rigorous methods and design:** You must show that your chosen study design will produce robust results and that you will provide data and methods so that others can reproduce your findings. Key issues are randomization, blinding, choice of outcome measure, optimizing measurement of the outcome, pre-specified statistical analysis, and adequate sample size and power.

3. **Consideration of sex and other relevant biological variables:** You need to show that you have considered demographic and other variables that may affect the outcomes of your study. These might include age, race, sex, co-morbidities, diet, circadian factors, and drug therapy. Always address the question of sex, reviewers look for it.

4. **Authentication of key biological or chemical resources:** You must show that you will regularly authenticate antibodies, cell lines, assays, and other experimental resources that may change over time.

The components of the rigor and reproducibility requirements were already an obvious part of a good grant, but now you must address them specifically and reviewers must check a box indicating that you have done so (2,3). Your discussion about rigor and reproducibility must fit into your 12 pages of science; some people use a separate paragraph entitled "rigor and reproducibility" to address the topics, others weave them into existing sections. For example, in the Approach section you can call out components of your design with the words "rigor" or "reproducibility." For example, *To ensure a rigorous design and reproducible findings we have chosen a sample size of...* The advantage of a separate paragraph is that the reviewer cannot miss it.

Summary

1. Think like a reviewer; ask yourself *so what?*

2. Perfect your Specific Aims before you write the rest of the grant.

3. Have a new and important question.

4. The goal of the Significance section is to sell your grant not to review the world literature.

5. Have a statistician as a co-investigator.

6. Have a clear, reproducible power and sample size section.

7. Use the Limitations/Pitfalls section to preempt reviewer questions but don't shoot yourself in the foot.

Resources

1. PSPower is a software program for calculating power and sample size that you can download for free.
   http://biostat.mc.vanderbilt.edu/wiki/Main/PowerSampleSize.
   The citation is Dupont WD, Plummer WD: Power and Sample Size Calculations: A Review and Computer Program, Controlled Clinical Trials 1990; 11:116-28.

2. Guidance on rigor and reproducibility in NIH applications.
   https://www.nih.gov/research-training/rigor-reproducibility/updated-application-instructions-enhance-rigor-reproducibility

3. Frequently asked question about NIH's rigor and transparency requirements. http://grants.nih.gov/reproducibility/faqs.htm#4836

4. How to apply for NIH grants. http://grants.nih.gov/grants/how-to-apply-application-guide.htm

5. The Northwestern University Collaborative Learning and Integrated Mentoring in the Biosciences (CLIMB) website provides very useful information in a series of short webinars.
   http://www.northwestern.edu/climb/resources/written-communication/index.html

6. Advice on NIH career-development grants.
   http://www.niaid.nih.gov/researchfunding/traincareer/pages/advice.aspx

7. The Grant Application Writers Workbook. National Institutes of Health Version. Robertson JD, Russell SW and Morrison DC. Grant Writers Seminars and Workshops, LLC (2018). A useful book that covers all components of grant writing and submission.

Chapter 14
Writing a grant – career development grants

THERE ARE THREE MAJOR DIFFERENCES between K-award career development grants and standard RO1 grants: 1) a section "The Candidate"; 2) a career development plan; and 3) a mentor's statement. Before you apply for a K-award, look at examples of successful applications to see how others designed their proposals.

The candidate

Your goal for this section is to tell a story that summarizes your training and success and describes your vision for your career. Toot your own horn; tell the reviewers about your research training, your mentor, your collaborations, your research interests and goals, your achievements, your commitment to an academic career, the support you have, your integration into a great environment, your training needs, and your future vision.

Career development plan

The career development plan is not a formality: Many candidates mistakenly believe that the career development plan is a formality that only requires a generic outline saying you will do a few courses and attend some lab meetings and grand rounds. That is a big mistake – many K-award applications fail because of a poor career development plan, not because of weak science.

The plan must be tailored to your career: You must tailor your career development plan specifically to your career. To show this clearly, spell out what skills you already have, identify some that are important for your future career but are missing from your portfolio, and describe how the K-award training would remedy that deficiency. Reviewers cannot infer what you do not spell out. For example, a candidate planning to do clinical research and one planning to do epidemiologic research need different training – yet both might believe that they will more than fulfill the expectations for training by obtaining a Master of Public Health (MPH) degree. Both should spell out how specific components of the MPH program will help them develop independence. Spell out your goals – both for your career and for your training program and show how they fit together.

The plan must be congruent with your career: Reviewers need a clear picture of your career goals; a vague description – *to be a physician-scientist* – is not adequate. Reviewers must also see that your training plan is congruent with your career goals. For example, if you are to be a bench scientist, you need to describe a program that provides the training you need to be successful bench scientist. How will an MSCI help you become a bench scientist? If you already have a PhD, how will a course in basic laboratory techniques add to your skills?

The plan must integrate with your research: Ideally, you will learn from both formal and informal training. If the formal training diverges from your research, explain the reasons clearly. For example, if you don't have a microbiome component in your studies but you propose microbiome training, you should convince the reviewer that this training will help you. It is useful to integrate your career development plans with practical experience in your research. For example, if you are taking a statistics course, explain the type of statistics you will use in your studies and show that, with mentorship, you will design and analyze those studies. A useful way to illustrate this integration is a time-line that integrates your career development and research plan. It is important for reviewers to understand which parts of the research plan you will actually perform. For example, if you propose a project that includes proteomics, clarify if you will learn to perform the proteomic studies and analyze the data, or if you will send your samples to a fee-for-service core laboratory. It makes sense to spend two years learning hands-on proteomics if this will be your future career. It does not make sense if you are planning a career with proteomics as one of many assays you will use.

Problems with the career development plan: Here are some examples of recurring criticisms of career development plans.

- *One of the didactic courses is Principles of A but it is unclear why A is important to the candidate's future career plans.*
- *Much of the proposal focuses on z, a new direction for the applicant, but there no training related to z.*
- *It is unclear how the career development plan will facilitate the applicant developing into an independent investigator and leader in the field.*
- *The career development plan is a timeline and a list of activities rather than having clear goals with a rationale and plan for obtaining them.*
- *The career development plan is a list of meetings the candidate would usually attend anyway with some courses interspersed.*
- *The career development plan is not integrated with the project; the candidate is doing two statistics course but a statistician will perform all the analyses.*
- *The candidate already has extensive training and it is unclear what the proposed training will add.*

The mentor and co-mentor's statement (letter)

Your mentor's letter is a critical component of your application and it should cover several key points listed below, not necessarily in this order.

1. *Why the mentor is your mentor and how he or she has already mentored you.*
   Reviewers want to know that your stated mentor(s) are indeed true mentors and not just placeholders on your application.

2. *The mentor is a successful scientist and has NIH funding.*
   Reviewers demand strong mentors; a K-quality mentor must have a strong reputation, current NIH funding, and proof of successful mentorship. Such a mentor is almost always at the level of Associate Professor or higher (Chapter 2).

3. *Why the mentor thinks you are a great candidate.*
   The mentor needs to tell the reviewers that because of your achievements, attitude, commitment, talent, and training you are worth investing in.

4. *Why the mentor thinks your proposed science is great.*
   By describing your science, the mentor demonstrates involvement and can also reinforce how your project and training plan integrate to advance your career.

5. *How the mentor helped design the training plan that will take you to independence.*
   Again, the mentor needs to show familiarity with your training plan and say why it is a great plan.

6. *How the mentor will help train and mentor you.*
   The mentor's plan to mentor you should be very specific and describe lab meetings and weekly one-on-one meetings, and discuss what those meetings will achieve and how the mentor will monitor your progress. The mentor's plan should include not only science but also grant applications, papers, career advancement to independence, and networking.

7. *How the mentor will evaluate your progress.*
   Reviewers like to see tangible goals (e.g., 2 papers a year, attend a scientific meeting together once a year, meet 3 leaders in the field, and submit an RO1 in year 3). The mentor should describe your mentoring committee, how often it meets, and how it assists in evaluating and guiding your progress.

8. *How your career will differentiate from that of the mentor.*
   If your project overlaps with your mentor's interests (which usually is the case), the mentor has to convince reviewers that you have an independent area of interest that will allow you to differentiate independently.

9. *Resources that the mentor will place at your disposal.*
   Reviewers know that K-grants do not provide enough funding for you to perform your research. They want assurance from your mentor that you will

have the resources (supplies, equipment, technicians, nursing support) you need.

10. Institutional resources that the mentor will help you access.
Most institutions have financial and mentoring resources to help develop scientists. Your mentor should describe these resources and how they will benefit you.

11. A clear path forward to independence.
Reviewers want to see the R award on the horizon; your mentor must paint that picture.

Problems with the mentor's letter

You might think that all mentors know how to write a strong letter for a K-award. That is not the case. Don't be afraid to offer to help construct and edit the mentor's statement. Make sure it covers all 11 points. If you have more than one mentor, they can write a joint letter; however, make sure they delineate exactly what role each will fill. Make sure your mentor's letter is concordant with your career plan; it looks bad if you say you will meet once a week, but your mentor says you will meet every two weeks. (You should meet once a week.) I have seen the following criticisms of mentors' letters:

- *does not describe a specific plan for the individual.*
- *the letter is generic.*
- *no specifics are provided about the mentoring plan.*
- *the applicant will be a pair of hands in the mentor's lab.*
- *no long-term goals are delineated.*
- *no progress milestones are provided.*
- *there is no monitoring of progress.*

Letters of support

Letters of support from collaborators and consultants must state their qualifications, their enthusiasm for you and the project, how they will contribute to both the science and your career development, and the resources they will make available to you. You should have a real Mentoring Committee (Chapter 5) that has met and provided a letter (signed by all) that describes their enthusiasm for you, the advisory roles they will fill, the frequency and format of meetings, and what steps they will take to guide you. Evidence that you have an ongoing relationship with a mentoring committee is much more compelling than a description of a future relationship that will only occur if you get the grant. You need letters from directors of your Department and Division. These letters must express great enthusiasm for you and your career, guarantee protected time, and describe institutional resources that will help you. Your mentor should work on these letters so that they are not generic. A letter of support from a senior scientist outside your institution who knows you and can vouch for your potential is also useful.

Timeline

Every grant application should have a timeline, but for career development applications the timeline should illustrate not only scientific but also training and career development goals. Your timeline must make sense; in the example below, you will see that in Aim 1 IRB approval is taking two years and data analysis has started before approval. If you have room, write some text to accompany the timeline and weave your training and research activities goals into a time-based narrative that plans your progress.

Example Career Award Timeline					
	Year 1	Year 2	Year 3	Year 4	Year 5
Mentorship					
Weekly meetings	X	X	X	X	X
6 monthly Mentorship Committee	X	X	X	X	X
Didactic Coursework					
MSCI	X	X			
Genetics 101 XYZ			X		
Annual Lukewarm Spring Meeting	X	X	X	X	X
Research					
Aim 1: To...					
Obtain IRB	X	X			
Data analysis	X	X	X		
Writing MS			X	X	
Aim 2: To...					
R01 Preparation				X	X

Summary

1. Look at successful career development grant applications.

2. The career development plan section of your grant is critically important; spend time on it.

3. You need a clear rationale for your training plan.

4. Your training plan must be congruent with your current skills and future career plans.

5. Your mentor must be K-quality and write a detailed mentoring statement. You should help edit this.

Resources

1. Advice about NIH career-development grants.

http://www.niaid.nih.gov/researchfunding/traincareer/pages/advice.aspx

2. Advice about mentored (K) career-development grants. http://www.niaid.nih.gov/researchfunding/traincareer/pages/mentorK.asp x

3. How to apply for NIH grants (specifically see the pdf with instructions for career development awards). http://grants.nih.gov/grants/how-to-apply-application-guide.htm

4. The Grant Application Writers Workbook. National Institutes of Health Version. Robertson JD, Russell SW and Morrison DC. Grant Writers Seminars and Workshops, LLC (2018). A useful book that covers all components of grant writing and submission.

5. A set of slides by Bill Hay that describes how to apply for a K-award. https://www2.aap.org/sections/perinatal/ONTPDFiles/PDFs/Tonse%20Final%20K%20grant%20applications.pdf.

6. Lindman BR, Tong CW, Carlson DE, Balke CW, Jackson EA, Madhur MS, Barac A, Abdalla M, Brittain EL, Desai N, Kates AM, Freeman AM, Mann DL. NIH career development awards for cardiovascular physician-scientists: recent trends and strategies for success. J Am Coll Cardiol. 2015;66(16):1816-1827. PMID: 26483107.

Chapter 15
Writing a grant – the non-scientific components

I WISH SUBMITTING A GRANT was as easy as emailing 12 pages of science, an abstract, and specific aims. Unfortunately not. You have to submit many other sections (1). In addition to being a scientist, you will be your own secretary, supervisor, and accountant. Leave plenty of time to complete these sections and do them well.

Deadlines

Many institutions have an internal deadline that falls approximately 2 weeks before the NIH submission deadlines (3 times a year for RO1s – February, June, and October) so that institutional administrators can approve your proposal and its budget. Usually, for internal deadlines you can submit a nearly final draft of the science (that you can continue to edit), but the budget must be final and you cannot change it without institutional re-approval. NIH deadlines are inflexible except if you (PI of the grant) have a death in the family, are seriously ill, or serve on an NIH study section in the two months before or after the date of submission. You can claim a two-week extension for those reasons. Late submissions are not preapproved. You send a cover letter with your application explaining why it is late and NIH decides whether or not it is accepted (2).

Work with a grants management specialist

Most research-intense institutions have grants management specialists to help you prepare and submit your grant. If your institution does not provide such support, you are in a poor environment for scientific success. Meet the grants manager several months before you plan to submit to identify internal deadlines and decide how the two of you will assemble the grant. Ideally, you will be responsible for the science and the sections described below, and the grants manager for the institutional forms and approvals, budget, face page, and assembling the grant for electronic submission. A knowledgeable and efficient grants manager is a wonderful asset.

Assembling the whole grant

It is a formidable task to assemble an NIH grant for the first time. In addition to the science sections (Abstract (30 lines), Introduction to Application (1 page, only for resubmissions), Specific Aims (1 page), Research Strategy (12 pages), and Bibliography) there are several other components (2).

Biosketches

Reviewers must answer the following questions about the investigators. Are the PI and collaborators well suited to the project? For early career investigators – do they have the appropriate expertise? For established investigators – have they been productive? For the research team – does the team bring together the necessary expertise to perform the studies?

Reviewers find the answers to these questions in the investigators' biosketches. Therefore, each investigator should tailor the personal statement section to highlight collaboration and expertise relevant to the specific proposal (Chapter 21). If you want to edit a co-investigator's biosketch to emphasize collaboration or expertise, do so in track changes and send the edited version back to your co-investigator for approval.

Project narrative section

This section used to be called the Public Health Statement. It consists of three sentences (a strict maximum) that summarize the relevance of the project for a lay audience in plain language. This short blurb becomes public for funded grants.

Budget

Direct and indirect costs: A grant has direct costs and indirect costs (3). Direct costs are the actual costs. Indirect costs are also called Facilities and Administrative (or F&A) costs and are informally called "institutional overhead." NIH pays universities these indirect costs (calculated as a percentage of your direct costs) to cover things like lights, water, libraries, and so on. Your grants manager will calculate the indirect costs for your budget.

Modular or detailed budget? NIH allows you to submit a modular budget (requiring few details and described in modules of $25,000) if your total direct costs are less than $250,000 a year. On the other hand, you cannot request more than $500,000 a year in direct costs without discussing the proposal with NIH. Most budgets are between $250,000 and $500,000 a year and require a non-modular (i.e., detailed) budget. Your chances of getting a grant are not affected by the size of the budget. Reviewers examine the science, score it, and then discuss if the budget is appropriate. A modular budget may seem attractive to you because it is simpler, but you will still need to construct a detailed budget for your own use (and some institutions require it for internal review).

Constructing the budget: When I start my budget, I first draft a detailed budget justification and then I ask my grants manager to enter the corresponding dollar amounts on a spreadsheet. As the grant evolves, I tweak the budget (and the justification) accordingly. NIH does not allow a built-in annual increase for inflation, so it is easiest to spread the costs evenly over 5 years (i.e., divide the direct costs for the total grant equally over 5 years). Recently, NIH has routinely reduced the budgets for new grants. Consequently, some game the system and overestimate the budget a little to offset the inevitable cut. Also, some ICs have been routinely cutting 5-year applications to 4 years. This is less likely to happen if you are a new investigator.

Budget justification

NIH designates the following subheadings in the budget justification:
A) Senior/Key Personnel
B) Other personnel
C) Equipment
D) Travel
E) Participant/Trainee Support Costs
F) Other direct costs (3).

A and B. Personnel: The personnel section has 2 subsections: A) Senior/Key Personnel are co-investigators who provide effort (i.e., the grant pays part of their salaries); B) Other Personnel are technicians, nurses, post doctoral students and others who have effort on the grant. NIH calculates effort in calendar months; in other words, 10% effort is 1.2 calendar months. For each person you provide a paragraph indicating the amount of effort devoted to the grant, what they will do, and why their contribution is important. For example:

Senior/Key Personnel

Mary Smith, M.D., Principal Investigator (4 calendar months effort with salary). As PI Dr. Smith will supervise all the activities of this project including the interaction between clinical and MRI experiments, study approaches, assessment of the progress as well as addressing potential experimental and technical problems, interpretation of data and submission of manuscripts.

Other Personnel

John Green, MSc., Database manager (0.6 calendar months effort with salary) Mr. Green is a database manager trained in statistics with experience in clinical database construction and management. He has assisted with the design of the study and will advise regarding final study design and will oversee the maintenance and quality of clinical databases and assist with the extraction of data for analysis.

As a general rule, the more effort someone has on a grant the more closely reviewers will scrutinize it. As PI, you should not request all your support from a single grant. As a beginning PI, you can usually ask for 50% effort (and perhaps more if you can justify it); an established PI would usually ask for 30%

or less. For each person it is important that the effort you request matches the tasks to be done. If you request too little effort for someone who will obviously do a lot of work, reviewers will criticize your budget (and your ability to do the study). Also, be careful about asking for support for individuals who are TBA (to be announced), particularly if they will fill important roles. If an important position on your grant is empty, it suggests absent expertise and potential vulnerability.

C. Equipment: Equipment is defined as an item costing $5,000 or more. You can buy less expensive pieces of equipment as part of your supplies. You must justify why you need to buy a particular piece of equipment by showing that you do not already have reasonable access to it and that its use will be dedicated to the grant. You do not always need a quote, but it is helpful include it. For example:

Equipment

We request $8,250 for the purchase of a -80 freezer in year 1. The study will generate approximately 800 samples that need to be stored at low temperatures to prevent oxidation. The PI has no access to an existing freezer for these samples. The price of $8,250 was quoted by XY Company (quote number 123, dated 2.10.2017) for an 18 cubic foot HyperCool -80 freezer. The freezer will be used exclusively for the current proposal.

D. Travel: It is reasonable to request funding to attend a national meeting. For example:

Travel

Funds are requested for the PI to attend a scientific meeting once a year to present findings and learn about advances in the field. = 1 trip @ $1500 = $ 1500/year

E. Participant/trainee support costs: This section is not applicable to the types of grants you are likely to apply for. It applies to institutional applications to train scientists.

F. Other direct costs

Materials and supplies: Itemize the broad categories of supplies (animals, lab supplies, cells, reagents and chemicals, and clinical supplies) that you will need and their dollar amount. For expensive categories it is useful to justify your estimate. For example:

Supplies

Patient food costs

In Aim 3 patients will purchase food they might not normally purchase for the high salt and low salt periods. We have found that adherence to a modified diet is greatly enhanced if patients are provide with resources to purchase foods for the menus prescribed. We budget $5 per day of altered diet x 112 days x 22 patients = $12,320/5 year = $2,464/year

Publication costs: You should budget for publication costs. Many journals have page charges. If your charges are reasonable they will be accepted without question, but if they are unusually high you must justify them. For example:

Publication Costs

We estimate that we will publish 2 papers a year. Our most frequent target journal is the Journal of Latest Imaging; this journal charges $1000 per paper and $1000 per color 3D figure – an essential presentation mode for studies of the type we will perform. We estimate publication costs of $3000 per paper and $6,000 per year.

Consultant costs: Consultants provide expertise, often for a fee, but sometimes for free, and do not have person months of effort on the budget. They are often external advisors who provide specific expertise for a short period of time. For example, a dietician might provide 2 days of consultation to help you set up diets. In your budget justification you should provide details about the number of days for consultation, the rate of compensation, and travel, accommodation, and meal costs (or a *per diem*). Sometimes individuals from your own institution might be consultants on your grant; this usually arises when you need to show senior expertise in a particular area, but the individual is too well funded and has no effort to devote to your grant. Designating such people as consultants (without compensation) allows you to include their expertise (and biosketches) in your grant. Consultants should write a letter of support (usually you draft it) that details what they will do for your grant.

Other direct costs: This is often one of the most expensive sections of the budget and it includes laboratory tests, patient re-imbursement, animal housing, and procedures you will perform for research. Organize the section with subheadings so that reviewers can understand where the costs come from. Under each heading, provide concrete numbers. These numbers must match with your science (e.g., Aim 1 will study 100 subjects x 4 CBC tests@ at $5 = $2000.

Facilities and equipment

Reviewers must answer the following questions about the environment. Will the scientific environment contribute to the likelihood of success? Do the investigators have the institutional support, equipment, and other resources they need to perform the proposed work? Are there unique strengths in the environment? Reviewers find these answers in your description of the studies and also in two separate sections: "Equipment" and "Facilities."

The Equipment section describes large pieces of equipment (usually owned by the institution) that you will use. For example, MRI machines, machines in the genetics or flow cytometry cores etc.

The Facilities section often starts with a paragraph that describes why the environment is great for the performance of the grant. This is followed by subheadings:

- *Laboratory*: describe the laboratories where you will do the studies, their size and location, and the equipment they have.

- *Animals:* describes where the animals will come from, where they will be housed, and the animal and veterinary facilities available. If you don't have animals, enter NA.

- *Clinical*: describe the source of patients (e.g., clinics) and where the studies will be done. For example, if appropriate, you would have a paragraph describing the CRC resources.

- *Computer*: describe computers you and the co-investigators have as well as your institution's network and IT resources.

- *Office*: describe your office size and location and discusses proximity to other investigators and laboratories or clinical sites.

- *Other Resources*: describe any other resources that will support your study (e.g., institutional Centers and Cores, statistical resources, bioengineering, machine shop, databases, CTSA resources). It is easiest to cut and paste this section from one of your mentor's grant applications and edit it.

Human Subjects and Clinical Trials Information

NIH requirements for human subjects' information changed in 2018 with the introduction of what is known as "Forms E." These requirements (1) are complex, confusing, and have increased the workload of clinical investigators submitting grants substantially. There are 5 Sections. If your grant includes more than one study you must submit a separate study record for each.

Section 1. Basic information

Are human subjects involved? If your study involves humans, or data or specimens from humans, you must check "Yes" in the "Humans Subjects Involved" box. If the answer is "no" you can stop here. Remember even if you never recruit a human subject and use de-identified data, you must check "yes" to the human subjects question. Confusion can arise because IRBs sometimes use the term "non-human subjects studies" to describe studies that use de-identified information and are exempt from Federal regulation.

Is your study is exempt from Federal regulations? There are 8 categories of possible exemption (4), but in reality only three are relevant: #1 (research conducted in an educational setting involving normal education practices); #2 (research using educational tests, surveys, interviews, or observations of public behavior unless identifiable and pose risks); and #4 (research involving the collection or study of existing data or specimens that are publicly available, or if the information is recorded so that subjects cannot be identified).

NIH-defined clinical trial? You will also be asked 4 questions to determine if your studies include a clinical trial (as defined by NIH): 1) Does the study involve human participants? 2) Are the participants prospectively assignment to an intervention? 3) Is the study designed to evaluate the effect of an intervention on the participants? 4) Is the effect that will be measured a health-related biomedical or behavioral outcome? If you answer yes to all four questions your study meets the NIH definition of a clinical trial. In other words, a study that assigns one child to watch a TV cartoon to see if the child keeps quiet during the show meets the definition.

The NIH further defines a Phase III clinical trial as follows: "a broadly based prospective clinical investigation, usually involving several hundred or more human subjects, for the purpose of evaluating an experimental intervention in comparison with a standard or controlled intervention or comparing two or more existing treatments." However, the "clinical trial" paperwork requirements for NIH relate to all NIH-defined clinical trials not just phase III trials.

If you answered "yes" to all 4 clinical trial questions you must complete all the subsequent sections (i.e., Sections 2-5); if you answered "no" to any of the 4 questions you do not need to complete sections 4 and 5.

Section 2. Study population characteristics

2.1 Conditions and focus of study
In this subsection you will enter a few MeSH subheadings to describe the area of research, similar to the keywords you select when you submit a paper to a journal

2.2 Eligibility criteria and 2.3 Age limits
In the text box type or paste your inclusion and exclusion criteria. Next (2.3) enter the age limits for your study.

2.4 Inclusion of women, minorities and children
Upload a pdf of your text (5). Clinical research must reflect the composition of the overall US population (51% women and 31% minorities) and not the local population where you plan to conduct the study. Describe the makeup of your study population, the rationale for this selection, and proposed outreach programs for recruiting. You must include the appropriate numbers of women and minorities unless you can provide a compelling scientific reason not to do so (e.g., you are studying prostate cancer). Remember, including men and women in your study is not the same as considering sex as a biological variable (one of

the areas you must address for rigor and reproducibility) (Chapter 13). If your study is an NIH-defined Phase III clinical trial, you must include plans for how sex and race will be taken into consideration in the design and analysis of the study in Section 2.4.

NIH requires you to include children (defined as individuals under the age of 18 years) in all clinical research unless you can provide a compelling scientific reason to exclude them. Children are usually excluded from clinical studies focused on adults because their physiology and disease pathogenesis and treatment is substantially different – a compelling scientific reason. The regulations regarding research in children and adults differ. If you do include children, you must make sure your human subjects section that describes recruitment, protection of vulnerable populations, risks and benefits, and procedures for obtaining consent includes the details relevant to performing research in children.

2.5 Recruitment and retention plan
Attach a pdf that explains where and how you plan to recruit and retain subjects.

2.6 Recruitment status
This is a self-explanatory drop-down menu that describes the current status of your study (e.g., not recruiting yet).

2.7 Study timeline
Attach text or a figure that shows a projected timeline. Do not use specific dates.

2.8 Enrollment of first subject
Enter the projected date of enrollment for your first subject into the dropdown menu.

Inclusion enrollment report
If human subjects are involved in your studies, you must fill out an inclusion enrollment report unless your study is exempt under exemption #4 (i.e., you are using publicly available or de-identified data.) The inclusion enrollment report breaks your recruitment numbers down by ethnicity, race, and sex.

Section 3. Protection and monitoring plans

3.1 Protection of human subjects
1. Risks to human subjects. In *subsection 1a.* describe the overall study design, the population, and how you will randomize or select study subjects. In *subsection 1b.* describe the research procedures, what data and specimens you will collect, how they will be stored, managed, and protected, and who will have access to protected information. Describe the risks to individuals, including risks from procedures and loss of privacy, and their likely frequency and potential seriousness. If there are alternative

treatments or procedures that you could perform, describe the rationale for what you propose to do.

2. *Adequacy of protection against risks:* This section is organized in the subsections below.

> *a. Informed consent and assent:* Describe how you will obtain informed consent. Include details about who will obtain consent and how consent will be documented. If you will include vulnerable populations or children you must include relevant details.
>
> *b. Protections against risk:* Describe how you will protect participants from risk (examples of protections include the expertise of the investigators, performing the study on the CRC, screening procedures to protect individuals etc.), and how confidentiality will be protected. If there are likely to be incidental findings (e.g., you will do CTs for coronary artery calcium and are likely to find incidental lung nodules), describe how you will handle those.
>
> *c. Vulnerable subjects:* If relevant to your study, explain the rationale for including vulnerable populations such as children, prisoners, and pregnant women. Such populations require additional protection against risk and you must describe how you will do that.

3. *Potential benefits of the proposed research to research participants and others:* Describe any benefits to participants (often there are none), the benefits to society (how the new knowledge will potentially advance care), and why the risks are reasonable considering the potential benefits. You should not consider subject reimbursement a benefit to participants.

4. *Importance of the knowledge to be gained:* Discuss the importance of the knowledge that will be gained and how this justifies the risks involved.

3.2 Is this a multi-site study using the same protocol?
If you check "yes," you are expected to use a single IRB.

3.3 Data and safety monitoring plan (DSMP)
If you have human subjects, you must have a data safety monitoring plan (DSMP), even if you do not propose an NIH-defined clinical trial (6). Your plan must include details about how you will maintain confidentiality and protect data, and how you will define and report adverse events (AEs) and serious adverse events (SAEs). In addition, you should describe how AEs will be detected (e.g., by patient report, questionnaire etc.), who will collect them (e.g., investigators, nurse), and who will be notified (e.g., IRB, FDA, CRC). Your plan must also provide details about safety monitoring. NIH states that "a variety of types of monitoring may be anticipated depending on the nature, size, and

complexity of the clinical trial. In many cases, the principal investigator would be expected to perform the monitoring function." In other words, not all NIH-defined clinical trials need a data safety monitoring board (DSMB) although all need a DSMP. It is up to you to decide the level of monitoring that is appropriate. If there is no intervention, and the biggest risks are those of loss of privacy and the dangers of venipuncture, you can say that adverse events will be monitored at the weekly lab meeting. For example:

> The proposed studies are low risk since they involve only the administration of a questionnaire and a blood draw. The principal investigator proposes to review the data and adverse events weekly and to forward those to the IRB, if warranted. During the conduct of the study, any serious adverse event related to the study will be reported to the IRB within 24 hours. Should the risk-benefit of the study change, the principal investigator will make alterations to the procedures of the study and submit them to the IRB.

For a more complex study, e.g., administration of a low-risk, FDA-approved drug to healthy subjects, you might consider including a Safety Officer (a local colleague not involved with the study) who will review the protocol and adverse event reports and make recommendations to you (and the IRB) as part of your data safety monitoring plan. For clinical studies that have higher risk, and for phase III clinical trials, a DSMB is appropriate. You need not name individuals but you should describe characteristics of the type of people who will serve on the DSMB.

3.4 Will a data and safety monitoring board (DSMB) be appointed for this study?

You must answer this question if your study is an NIH-defined clinical trial; answering is optional for other studies involving human subjects.

3.5 Overall structure of the study team

For NIH-defined clinical trials attach a pdf that describes the organizational structure of the study team, including administrative and laboratory sites. Do not include personal biographic information about investigators; describe their roles.

Section 4. Protocol synopsis

4.1 Brief summary

In the text box enter an abstract that describes the study, including its primary and secondary outcomes in fewer than 5000 characters. No Figures or Tables are allowed in the abstract and some Word characters do not copy and paste into the textbox.

4.2 Study Design

4.2a Narrative study description: You describe your protocol in fewer than 32,000 characters. Describe important baseline considerations (e.g., matching), randomization, the intervention (what, when, why, how, quality control etc.), procedures, the outcomes (what, when, why, how measured, quality control etc.), and data collection and storage. Again, this is a text box entry – simple text works best.

4.2b Primary purpose: Choose the most appropriate word that describes your study from the pull down list (e.g., treatment, prevention, etc.). If none of the options is appropriate select the "other" option and enter a few words to describe your purpose.

4.2c Interventions: Enter or select the intervention(s) you will use from the pull down list (e.g., drug, device, dietary supplement etc.)

4.2d-g: These sections are self explanatory and you select the option that describes your design (e.g., Phase 1, parallel, masked participants and investigators, randomized).

4.3 Outcome measures
For each outcome measure fill in the fields that ask you for the name of the outcome measure; whether it is primary, secondary or other; when it will be measured, and a brief description of the outcome measure.

4.4 Statistical design and power
Attach a pdf that provides your sample size calculation and statistical methods. This sample size and statistics text was previously a standard part of the 12 pages of science (Chapter 13); your science section will now only summarize these and refer the reader to this section for the details.

4.5 Subject participation duration
Fill in the time it will take for each subject to complete the study.

4.6 Will the study use an FDA-regulated intervention
The term FDA-regulated intervention includes prescription drugs, approved devices, and investigational drugs and devices. If you tick "yes" to the box, you will be asked to append (subsection 4.6a) a pdf indicating where you will get the drug, and how it will be administered. Also you will be asked to indicate the investigational new drug (IND) status of the drug. IRBs will generally not require an IND for most FDA-approved drugs used in research if: the work does not seek to change the indication or advertising for the drug; the drug is used in the same doses and route of administration, in the same patient population, and with the same likely risk profile as the marketed product. If you or your IRB is uncertain you can apply to the FDA for an IND exemption (7).

4.7 Dissemination plan
Load a pdf that says at least 3 things: 1) that the study will be registered on clinical trials.gov and the results posted there; 2) that your consent form will include a statement that says that the results of the study will be posted on clinical trials.gov; 3) that your institution has internal policies in place to ensure clinical trial registration and posting of results.

Section 5. Other clinical trial-related attachments

If your funding opportunity announcement requires or permits attachments you can attach them here.

Vertebrate animals

If your grant includes studies in animals, you must cover the following three areas.

1. Describe procedures: Provide a description of the experimental procedures and describe the animals you will use (total number, sex, species, strains and ages).

2. Justifications: Explain why you could not do the research without using animals (e.g., why alternate cell models are inadequate) and justify the appropriateness of the species studied.

3. Minimization of pain and distress: Describe what distress you may cause the animals and what interventions you will put in place to minimize this (e.g., anesthesia, sedation, postoperative care).

Biohazards and select agent research

This section is not applicable to most grants; if needed, you can find instructions online. Biohazards are hazards such as organisms, toxins, radioactivity, dangerous chemicals, or recombinant DNA that pose a particularly significant risk to research personnel or the environment. Select Agents are biological agents and toxins identified by government bodies as having the potential to be a severe threat to public health and safety (e.g., ebola virus, ricin) (8).

Resource sharing plan

You must describe a reasonable plan to share your data (or explain why this is not feasible) if your application has direct costs of $500,000 or more in any year (9). A grant that develops model organisms must describe a plan for sharing the organism. Any NIH grant that generates large-scale human or non-human genomic data (e.g., genome wide association studies) must include a genomic data sharing plan.

Letter of support

If you are submitting an application for a mentored grant, you will require letters of support. Follow the instructions; the page limit for many grants is 6 pages for letters from collaborators, contributors, and consultants, and 6 pages for the Mentor's and Co-Mentors' Statement. For other grants (e.g., RO1s), you generally only need letters of support from consultants and co-investigators at other institutions. The letters delineate the person's expertise, what they will do for your grant, and how wonderful they think you and the grant are.

Multiple PD/PI leadership

For Co-principal investigator (Co-PI) grants, this section should describe the rationale for a multiple-PI approach, the governance and organizational structure of the project, communication plans, the process for making decisions, and procedures for resolving conflicts (10). A Co-PI grant must benefit from having two Co-PIs; each PI must have a clearly distinguishable area of expertise that is important for the success of the grant. For example, in a study of gene expression in asthma, one PI is expert in gene expression and the other in asthma. If such a situation is not present, Co-PI status is difficult to justify. Doing equal work, or requiring equal recognition, does not justify a Co-PI application. New Investigator and Early Stage Investigator status only applies to applications on which all Co-PIs qualify for this status. If you are a Co-PI on a funded grant, you lose your New Investigator status.

Cover letter

You do not need a cover letter unless you need to justify a late application. The assignment request form has supplanted the other purposes of the cover letter.

Assignment request form

You use the assignment request form to request assignment to particular institutes for funding consideration and to a particular study section for review (discussed next). You can also outline the expertise that reviewers of your grant will require (but you cannot suggest specific reviewers). You can ask (with reasons provided) that certain reviewers not be assigned your grant; such requests are unusual.

Which institute should you request? The Center for Scientific Review (CSR) handles grant submissions and assigns applications to a primary institute or center (IC) as the source for potential funding. CSR assigns based on the content of the grant and the focus of particular institutes. Your grant could be of interest to more than one institute and also assigned to a secondary institute. For example, a grant about heart disease in rheumatoid arthritis could be assigned to NHLBI (primary) and NIAMS (secondary). Grants assigned to more than one institute are said to have a better chance of funding because if the score is borderline, and the primary institute is unable to fund it, the secondary institute might. That has not happened in my personal experience. Different ICs have different paylines (the percentile above which grants are funded); for example, in 2016 the paylines for NHLBI and NCI were 14% and 10%, respectively (11). Talk to the POs (Chapter 16) of various institutes to decide which assignment is most appropriate and advantageous.

Which study section should you request? In addition to assigning your grant to an institute, CSR also assigns it to a study section. Your grant will have a better chance of success if a study section that is knowledgeable and sympathetic to a particular area of science reviews it. You must do some work to find out which study section is most appropriate for your grant. Study sections are organized under broader Integrated Review Groups (IRGs). Each IRG represents a general scientific area (e.g., cardiovascular and respiratory disease) and has several study sections. On the NIH website about study sections (12,13) you can enter key words and read about the focus of a particular study section to see if your grant is suitable for it. Also, the NIH RePORTER website (14) has a useful tool called Matchmaker. On the RePORTER home page, if you click on the Matchmaker button it will open a text box into which you paste your abstract. The tool will then search for the funded grant applications most similar to yours and tell you which IC funded them and which study section reviewed them. However, you should also speak to the PO or someone who has been on the study section to help you choose a study section. You can find a list of study section members online (15). Don't be scared to speak to people at your institution who have sat on a particular study section. Research the members of a study section and see what type of research they publish. You can often predict which person on a study section is likely to review your grant; make sure you cite appropriate references to show that you are aware of that individual's work.

Internal routing: Your institution has to sign off on your grant application. Usually, you have to submit the budget and a draft of the science approximately 2 weeks before the NIH deadline. Make sure you meet this deadline.

Final submission: You submit to NIH electronically. Your grants manager can help by lodging all the required sections for you, but before you hit the final button, print the entire document and read it over quickly. Look for figures that have moved, widows and orphans (single lines at the beginning or end of a page that are stranded), and formatting errors. Other than correcting errors, this is not the time to make minor editorial changes. Once you have submitted the grant you will receive a message that it was received, usually within an hour. You will also receive an email telling you about several errors; usually these are minor administrative or business details related to the ways certain forms were completed. Your grants manager can help you decide if these are true errors you need to fix; if so, you must do so before the grant deadline. Submitting a day or two early is prudent.

Summary

1. NIH deadlines are inflexible.

2. Submitting a grant is a complex process; start early, work with an experienced grants manager, and keep to a timeline.

3. The non-science parts of NIH grants are to some extent cut-and-paste and ticking of boxes, but make sure you do them well. Get examples from you mentor.

4. Start your budget early and prepare a detailed budget. You will not get the budget you ask for.

5. Give thought to which institute and study section are best for your application. Discuss this with the PO.

6. Submit a few days early.

Resources

1. This is the daunting application guide for NIH grants. If you scroll down to "Application Form Instructions (SF424 R&R- Version E)" you will see a "General Instruction" pdf (293 pages) and "Research (R) Instructions" pdf (143 pages). You should dip into these, but by far the easiest way to figure things out is to look at recently submitted grants and to work with a grants specialist.   https://grants.nih.gov/grants/how-to-apply-application-guide.htm

2. Information about NIH's policy for late submission of grants. http://grants.nih.gov/grants/policy/late_application_faq.htm

3. Information about budgets for NIH grants. http://grants.nih.gov/grants/how-to-apply-application-guide/format-and-write/develop-your-budget.htm

4. Describes research exempt from human subjects regulations. http://www.hhs.gov/ohrp/regulations-and-policy/regulations/45-cfr-46/index.html#46.101

5. Inclusion of Minorities and Women in Study Populations- Questions and Answers.   https://www.nhlbi.nih.gov/grants-and-training/policies-and-guidelines/inclusion-of-minorities-and-women-in-study-populations-questions-and-answers

6. Information about setting up a data safety monitoring board. http://www.nidcr.nih.gov/Research/ToolsforResearchers/Toolkit/DSMBGuidelines.htm

7. INDs and IND exemptions.
   https://www.fda.gov/Drugs/DevelopmentApprovalProcess/HowDrugsareD
   evelopedandApproved/ApprovalApplications/InvestigationalNewDrugIND
   Application/ucm362743.htm

8. A list of select agents.
   http://www.selectagents.gov/SelectAgentsandToxinsList.html

9. Data and resource sharing. http://grants.nih.gov/policy/sharing.htm

10. Information about multiple PI applications.
    http://grants.nih.gov/grants/multi_pi/overview.htm

11. Success rates of NIH applications by institute and other parameters.
    https://report.nih.gov/success_rates/index.aspx

12. Find the right study section.
    http://public.csr.nih.gov/StudySections/Pages/default.aspx

13. Researching NIH study sections.
    http://public.csr.nih.gov/StudySections/IntegratedReviewGroups/Pages/d
    efault.aspx

14. NIH RePORTER site (to use the Matchmaker tool).
    https://projectreporter.nih.gov/reporter.cfm

15. Study section rosters. http://public.csr.nih.gov/RosterAndMeetings/

16. The Grant Application Writers Workbook. National Institutes of Health
    Version. Robertson JD, Russell SW and Morrison DC. Grant Writers
    Seminars and Workshops, LLC (2018). A useful book that covers all
    components of grant writing and submission.

Chapter 16

Writing a grant – after you get your score

Interpreting the score

A few days after the study section has met, the impact score for your grant will appear on eRA Commons, and a few days after that you will receive an email telling you the score is available. Any numeric score is good; the worst outcome is "not discussed" (so-called "streamlined" but in truth triaged). Your immediate emotion will be elation if you have a score of 1 or 2 and despair if your grant was not discussed. If your grant was scored, look at your percentile and then look up the current payline for your institute. Some institutes publish their paylines for established and new investigators for different types of grants (1). Unfortunately, no matter how outstanding your score, you cannot be certain you will be funded. Generally, if you are better than the 10th percentile your chances of being funded are excellent; if you are an ESI the fundable payline can extend to the 20th percentile. The only way to get an idea whether your scored grant has a chance of being funded is to speak to the PO.

Speaking to the PO

The grant reviews (officially called summary statements, but unofficially called "pink sheets" by the oldtimers because they used to be on pink paper) will be available a few weeks after the score is posted. There is little point in arranging a call with the PO until you have read your summary statement. Even then, the PO often cannot give you a definite answer whether your grant will be funded. Your grant still has to proceed to the advisory council for that institute. Program officials make funding recommendations to the advisory council, which in turn makes recommendations to the institute director, who makes the final decision. Also, program staff may not know how much money will be available in that government fiscal year or grant cycle, so they may not know the paylines yet. Because of this, program staff can often only talk in generalities about the likelihood that you will be funded and you are left to interpret their heavily qualified adjectives (2).

Just-in-time requests

Every grant with a score of 40 or better receives an automated request for just-in-time (JIT) information. JIT information includes other support (active and pending support for key personnel), Institutional Animal Care and Use Committee (IACUC) documents if you have animal studies, and Institutional Review Board (IRB) certification if you have human studies. This JIT request does not mean that you will be funded. You should ignore the automated JIT request if you are uncertain if you will be funded. If NIH sends a second request for JIT information a month or two before the start date, that is a positive sign that you might be funded. But often you will not be certain if a grant will be funded or what its start date will be until your institution receives the notice of grant award (NOA), also sometime called a NOGA. Unfortunately, this means that sometimes you will have to go ahead and prepare to resubmit only to find out later that your original application was eventually funded (a happy outcome but nevertheless a waste of your time).

Not Funded – options

Remember, NIH receives thousands of applications (approximately 50,000 research project grant applications in 2015) and the review process is imperfect. If your grant is not funded you have three options: 1) appeal the review; 2) abandon the grant; and 3) resubmit.

1) Appeal the review

Although my usual first emotion is how stupid the reviewers were (and besides, they never even read it!), appeals are rare and seldom successful. The best outcome of an appeal is a re-review (which is fundamentally the same as a resubmission) (2). Differences of opinion are not grounds for appeal. But, if the reviewer was biased (aren't we all), had a conflict of interest, or made factual errors (don't we all) that could have altered the outcome, there could be grounds for appeal. I don't recommend even considering this route unless the reviewer was egregiously, obviously, and absolutely wrong, and even then I would probably resubmit with a quiet word to the PO to pass on to the SRO about the problematic reviewer.

2) Abandon the grant

If you grant is triaged and you cannot address the reviewers' comments, you may be wise to abandon the grant and start over. Everyone has a tendency to overreact initially, so delay a decision like this and discuss it with your mentor and PO. These days, you can resubmit a grant as many times as you have energy for (as a new submission under a different title if it has bounced twice), but realistically there is little point in wasting everyone's time (particularly yours). If you abandon a grant, it does not necessarily mean you abandon an idea. You can submit a new grant that uses the same preliminary data to address different questions.

3) Resubmit

Resubmitting a grant is not like resubmitting a paper. If a journal invites you to revise and resubmit a paper it is often a conditional acceptance; this is not the case with grants – in fact, you may get a worse score second time around. When you resubmit you must identify the major criticisms and answer them convincingly. Remember Red Auerbach's words: *It's not what you say, it's what they hear.* Approach your revision with the attitude that all the criticisms, even unfair, incorrect, and stupid ones, are your problem because you did not explain things clearly enough to the reviewer. Your resubmission starts with getting extra data that you need to answer questions and working on the Introduction (3).

Introduction: You get one extra page in a revised grant to address reviewers' comments. This page is called the Introduction. I start the Introduction by quoting examples of great things the reviewers said about the grant. (Reviewers always say something positive, even for applications they triage.) Then tell the reviewers how you have changed the application. Remember, just as when you revise a paper, you require diplomacy and you should not whine, grovel, or bite (Chapter 9). You identify reviewer criticisms (combining themes from different reviewers) and briefly paraphrase or quote these (in italicized text) and then say how you have dealt with them. As an example, here is part of the Introduction for a grant I recently resubmitted (the original was triaged).

INTRODUCTION

This is a revised submission of an application for which the review committee *"agreed that the significance of the study, if successful, is high since findings could advance mechanistic understanding of how salt regulates inflammation and blood pressure which could potentially lead to new therapeutics."* Additional key strengths included *the innovative MRI approach, strong PI and team, and superb environment.* The concerns the reviewers raised have been addressed as described below and additionally in the application.

Lack of key preliminary data in RA: We had presented extensive preliminary data in cells, animals, and humans to support the premise and feasibility. Reviewers requested studies in rheumatoid arthritis (RA) supporting the hypothesis. Accordingly, we have measured skin Na^+ by ^{23}Na MRI in 5 patients with RA and 8 controls without RA; the findings are in keeping in keeping with our hypothesis skin Na^+ is higher in RA and that higher skin Na^+ is associated with higher RA disease activity (See Preliminary Data and Fig x).

Preliminary data lacking – 1) ...that skin Na^+ can be reliably quantified; 2) to support technically challenging ^{23}Na MRI quantification of skin Na^+ content; 3) ...exactly where sodium is stored in the skin... : 1) We have performed additional studies in animals and humans (Figs x and y in the grant) that show... 2) We provide reproducibility data...

Revise, revise, revise

Previously, when you revised a grant you had to mark the revisions in the body of the grant, but now that is optional. I generally do not mark the revisions, but I do underline or bold phrases in the grant (often present previously) that reviewers missed and asked questions about. Your mentor and other internal reviewers must read your resubmission. There is a tendency to rush back in, and NIH sends new investigators their pink sheets as soon as possible to give them time to resubmit in the next cycle. Rushing back is a mistake; polish the product till it is glorious.

Summary

1. Unless you get a near-perfect score and percentile you cannot be certain your grant will be funded. Arrange (by email) a call with the PO after you have the summary statement.

2. The rebuttal (Introduction) must be positive, diplomatic, and authoritative.

3. Your mentor and other internal reviewers must review the resubmission.

4. Very good is not good enough, your resubmission must be perfect.

Resources

1. Information about the review and post review process. http://grants.nih.gov/grants/peer_review_process.htm

2. Kienholz ML, Berg JM. How the NIH can help you get funded. Oxford University Press 2014. This book provides an insider's view into the functioning of the NIH-grant funding mechanism.

3. Information about resubmitting an NIH grant. http://grants.nih.gov/grants/policy/resubmission_q%26a.htm

Chapter 17
Writing a grant – common mistakes

WE HAVE COVERED MANY COMMON GRANTWRITING MISTAKES in the previous chapters, but it is worth summarizing those that are most injurious.

Boring or trivial question

For reviewers to advocate for you, your question must be new, interesting, and important.

The rationale for the grant is not compelling

You may believe the world is flat, but unless you can back that up with well-argued suggestive evidence, you will not convince a reviewer.

Specific Aim depends on the success of previous Aim

Aims that depend on each other are fatal.

Rushing the grant

It takes a long time to write a successful grant – every component requires thought, reading, writing, revision, and editing. A lot of that time is spent thinking, reading, and evaluating Specific Aims. This intellectual process takes time. Once the Specific Aims are clear and tight, the rest of the grant is much easier to write.

Not getting internal reviews

Other people must read and criticize your grant. It is much easier for them to read one page of flawed Specific Aims than 12 pages of flawed grant. So, get reviews at the Specific Aims stage – before you write the body of the grant.

Rushing internal reviews

It is unfair to ask a reviewer to look over your grant a few days before it is due. To get the most out of your internal reviewers, you should have a final version of the grant ready for internal review a month or two before the deadline.

Not following instructions

The instructions for grant applications are not negotiable. The deadline is inviolate. The page limits are strictly enforced. If you apply in response to a specific request, your grant must be responsive to that request. There is no room for negotiation. If you are uncertain, email the PO to arrange a call to discuss whether your grant is responsive.

Science too complicated

A grant with too many Specific Aims, too many experiments, and too many variables is difficult to sell.

Style too complicated

Long, dense sentences and paragraphs that leave complex concepts unexplained predestine your grant to failure. However, reviewers may not tell you this is the reason. Few reviewers have the self-confidence to say they don't understand a grant. It is more likely they will nitpick at something more concrete that may seem trivial and fixable to you (e.g., Applicant did not adequately describe matching of the control group).

Irritating style

A reviewer's threshold for irritation is low. Abbreviations can be irritating, use them sparingly. Other sources of irritation include illegible figures and figure legends, no legend explaining what a figure means, typos, having the Specific Aims stated differently in different places, obvious cut-and-paste errors from another grant, and poor organization.

No power/sample size/statistician

Even basic science grants must discuss statistical power and sample size, and it is a rare grant that does not benefit from a statistical collaborator or consultant. A reviewer must understand your power calculation and be able to reproduce it with the information you provide.

Missing letters of support and other sloppiness

If you propose to use anything (e.g., a drug, an animal model, stored samples, a cohort of patients) that depends on the expertise or goodwill of someone outside the grant, you should get a letter of support from the person promising the resource. If you are relying heavily on the intellectual expertise of someone who is not a co-investigator, it is a good idea to make the person a consultant to the grant (often unpaid, but always with a letter of support and biosketch). Careless errors show sloppiness and antagonize reviewers.

Chapter 18
Reviewing grants – your first study section

Accept the invitation and prepare

At some point you are likely to be invited to be an *ad hoc* reviewer on an NIH study section. By this time your rank will likely assistant professor or higher and you will have at least one NIH grant. If you are not invited and want to volunteer you can send an email to the Enhancing Peer Review mailbox (ReviewerVolunteer@mail.nih.gov) with a sentence or two about your areas of expertise and a copy of your biosketch. Also, if you have not yet received an RO1 and want to experience the review process, you can join NIH's early career reviewer (ECR) program (1) that will train you to be a reviewer and allow you to sit in on some study section meetings. The scientific review officer (SRO) sends emails inviting *ad hoc* reviewers about six months before the study section meeting. It is almost always a good idea to accept an invitation to review for NIH. Not only do you meet the people who might review your future grants, but you learn about cutting-edge science. You also get an insider's view of how study sections review grants in your area. So unless you have already accepted an invitation from another study section, you should accept. You should read the guidelines for reviewers and watch a video about study section on the NIH website (2,3).

What happens after you accept the invitation?

Acceptance is not rescindable: After you've accepted the invitation, make sure to enter it on your calendar and block time in the preceding months to review the grants. Once you've accepted the invitation, only death and serious illness are reasonable excuses for defaulting.

Do you have conflicts of interest? The SRO will send you a list of the applicants, co-investigators, and their institutions and ask you if you have a conflict of interest with any of the applications. The SRO will ask you to declare your conflicts of interest again before, during, and after the meeting. If you inadvertently overlook a conflict of interest and discover it later, notify the SRO immediately.

What is a conflict of interest for NIH reviews? The conflict of interest document that you sign explains the NIH rules. To summarize, you should recuse yourself if you (or a significant other such as a spouse, child, or relative) have, have had, or intend to have, any of the following relationships with any of the key personnel or contributors to the application:

- a mentor or mentee relationship
- are from your current or previous institution
- co-authored a paper, applied for a grant together, or otherwise collaborated within the previous three years
- you serve in any capacity on the grant or other grants with the applicants, including membership of data safety monitoring boards
- you are applying for a job at their institution or they are applying for a job at yours

You should also recuse yourself if you have a personal conflict of interest (e.g., a strong dislike for a person), or a scientific conflict of interest (e.g., you are doing, or plan to do, the same work) (Chapter 27). I generally scan the list of names and if I recognize any of them I ask myself if there could be an appearance of a conflict of interest between myself and that person. If you are uncertain whether a particular relationship constitutes a conflict of interest, ask the SRO.

Reviewing the grants

Check your assignments: A few months before the meeting date you will receive an email from the SRO saying that the grants assigned to you are now available for review. You access the grants and submit your reviews electronically; you will need to sign on to the eRA (electronic research administration) NIH commons website and then go to the "internet assisted review" (IAR) section. There you will find the list of grants allocated to you and whether you are first, second, or third reviewer. There are also review forms and additional materials. Even though your reviews are only due in several months, take a quick look at all the grants you will review. Check for two things: first, did a conflict of interest escape you; second, are any of the grants so far out of your area of expertise that you cannot review them. It is far easier to ask the SRO to reassign a grant now than to ask two weeks before the meeting. Remember, you should not expect to review grants only in areas in which you are expert; general expertise in the area is acceptable, particularly if you are the second or third reviewer.

Reviewing the grants: Just as when you review a paper (Chapter 10), you have heavy responsibilities when you review a grant: to be conscientious, fair, and impartial and maintain confidentiality. It is overwhelming when you first see your electronic pile of assigned grants; tackle them one at a time. I start months before the meeting and spend an evening flipping through all the grants. Then I read one grant per evening. After I have spent an evening reading a grant, I spend the next evening rereading it and writing a draft of my review. Then I move on to the next grant. When I have finished, I look over them all again to make sure my calibration did not shift while I was reviewing.

After you have read the grant, formed your opinions, and are ready to write the review, download the review form from the "meeting materials" section of the IAR section on eRA Commons. Unlike reviewing a paper, you will have to provide numeric scores and short paragraphs or bullet points that justify your scores. NIH uses the "overall impact" score to determine which grants are funded, but you will also provide scores and accompanying text for the individual sections of the grant: Significance, Investigators, Innovation, Approach, and Environment. Let's deal with the scoring system first and then the individual sections.

The NIH scoring system: The possible scores for the grant and its subsections range from 1-9 with no fractions. Reviewers are encouraged to spread the scores across the range in order to avoid applications clumping in the 1-3 range. A good, medium-impact grant should score 5. The descriptors for numeric scores 1-9 are listed in Chapter 13.

Your numbers and text should be concordant and internally consistent: Your overall impact score – the score that really matters – should be consistent with at least some of your individual section scores. For example, if you give an overall score of 5, then at least some individual section scores should be 5 or worse. Similarly, you should not give an overall score of 2 if none of your subsection scores are 2 or better. The text accompanying each score is organized as bulleted strengths and weaknesses. The text you provide for each section should be consistent with your score for that section. For example, if you give a score of 4 for section but don't mention any weaknesses, the applicant will be confused (and indignant). Similarly, if you give a score of 2 (extremely strong with negligible weaknesses) to a section but you don't mention any strengths, or you mention some strengths but also several weaknesses, there will be a disconnect between your score and your text. Just as when you review a paper, use diplomatic, bland, and constructive words.

Overall impact: You provide an overall impact score and a paragraph to justify your score. The overall impact score is not the numeric average of your scores for the individual sections. Rather, it is your assessment of the overall likelihood that the work will have a sustained and powerful effect on the research field involved. NIH reports that the overall impact score tracks most closely with the score reviewers give to the Approach section of the grant. The text for the Overall section is often 8-20 lines long and is not bulleted. This text is not a summary of what the applicant proposes to do; it is a summary of the most important strengths and weaknesses of the grant that influenced your overall score. The text of the Overall section inevitably repeats some of the points you made in the bulleted strengths and weaknesses text for the individual sections.

Significance: Your review of the Significance section evaluates whether the question is important and whether the work is likely to advance the field significantly. In this section and the others, list the strengths and weaknesses in bullet points. You are not obliged to nitpick because you feel pressure to write something under the weaknesses heading; it is acceptable to write "No significant weaknesses," and for your section score to reflect that statement (a score of 1 or 2). The more you write under weaknesses, the worse you score should be.

Investigators: Is the PI well-qualified to perform the studies? Does the study team have the right mix of expertise and experience?

Innovation: Innovation is not the same as significance and is defined in Chapter 13. You ask the following questions. Does the grant challenge or shift the *status quo* using novel approaches? Does it use methods that have advantages over previous work? Could the grant bring advances to a broad field rather than just a narrow area?

Approach: This is the section reviewers accord the most weight. Are the methods sound? Do the experiments proposed make sense? Will the study design answer the question? Does the applicant consider alternative approaches and discuss potential outcomes intelligently? Remember, no one can design a study that another scientist believes is perfect. The studies do not have to be done the way you would do them, but they should not contain design errors. In my opinion, perhaps because readers can understand them more easily, clinical studies are criticized unfairly more often than basic science studies for trivial details in the Approach.

Environment: Does the investigator have the resources to do the study? Are there unusual intellectual or physical resources that facilitate the success of the study?

Additional Review Criteria

The review form will prompt you to select options from a pull-down menu for some sections of the grant (e.g., Protections for Human Subjects; Inclusion of Women, Minorities, and Children; Vertebrate Animals; Biohazards). Your review of these sections can factor into your score but review of the budget should not.

Submitting your reviews

Submit your reviews electronically through the IAR section of the eRA Commons website before the deadline. After the deadline, the status of reviews will change from "review" to "read," and you will be able to see the other reviewers' scores and reviews. It is important to read what others thought about the grants you reviewed, particularly if your scores are very different from theirs.

Study section meeting

Travel arrangements: The SRO will send you details about travel arrangements. You will need to book your flight through the NIH-designated travel agency. It helps to search for flights that suit you and request those. NIH will book your hotel and pay for it, but you will have to provide a credit card when you check-in to cover any additional costs. NIH gives you a flat fee for ground travel costs (taxi, parking etc.), a *per diem* for meals, and an honorarium of $200/day (not including travel days). The night before the meeting you should look over the grants you reviewed, particularly those for which you were the primary reviewer, and think about what you plan to say.

The meeting: Arrive 20 minutes before the meeting. You will enter a poorly ventilated, subterranean, windowless room in an urban hotel. There will be coffee available. Several NIH staff members will be sitting at the back of the room. There will be a large rectangular cramped seating arrangement with assigned seats. Find the seat with your name and get yourself organized. There will be a power strip for your computer, and a folder with the agenda, conflicts of interest, the order in which grants will be reviewed, and your score sheet. Introduce yourself to your neighbor on both sides, and when you get a chance (either before the meeting or during a break), introduce yourself to the chair of the study section, the SRO, and members of the study section that interest you – this is a chance to network. The meeting will start on time. The SRO will start the meeting by reviewing the rules and summarizing meeting procedures. Then there will be a process to "streamline" the applications. This is a euphemism for triaging proposals. The triaging process is based on the distribution of the scores that you and the other reviewers submitted online. If all the reviewers' scores for a particular application were uniformly below average, the application will be triaged. Those applications will not be discussed further, but the applicants receive the reviewers' written comments. Any reviewer can ask to discuss a grant that is slated for triage, but this is unusual. Once the the final list of grants is determined, the reviews start.

How grants are reviewed: The chair introduces each grant, and if you have a conflict with that grant, you leave the room. The chair then asks each of the 3 reviewers to provide a preliminary overall impact score (this is the score submitted in the written reviews). The primary reviewer (reviewer 1) then presents his or her review highlighting the strengths and weaknesses of the grant, followed by reviewer 2 and then reviewer 3. The chair then asks for reviewer comments on the Protections for Human Subjects; Inclusion of Women, Minorities, and Children; Vertebrate Animals; and Biohazards section. (Make sure you remember to note in your written review if the applications meets the criteria.) Then the whole group discusses the grant. After the discussion, the chair asks the 3 reviewers for their amended final impact score based on what they have discussed. The assigned reviewers' scores set the voting range; for example, if their scores are 1, 2, and 3, then the voting range for the entire group is 1 to 3. If you want to vote outside that range you should say that you are doing so and state your reason. For example, "I am scoring outside the range. I think this is a 4 because I heard several minor weaknesses in the discussion." You then record your score on your paper score sheet and usually also on an electronic score sheet (so take a laptop).

The chair then asks reviewers to comment on the budget. Don't nitpick; you don't have to criticize the budget. If you do so, you must suggest a concrete cuts (e.g., "I don't think they need two full-time nurses to recruit 30 patients, and I suggest cutting one of the nurses.")

Presenting your review: The primary reviewer has the toughest job. The written reviews are mostly bulleted strengths and weaknesses, whereas the primary reviewer presents a narrative. Although you will have internet access to the reviews you submitted, I find it easier to print my review to remind me what I thought. Do not read your written review. If you do so, the overall impact section and the subsequent sections will repeat many points, and you will repeat yourself. As primary reviewer, I usually start by saying, "This is an (insert appropriate adjective that matches the NIH score table, e.g., "outstanding" for a grant that you gave a score of 2) that addresses the problem of...." I then describe the significance of the problem followed by a brief paraphrase of the Aims of the grant. Then, I talk about the approach bringing in strengths and weaknesses followed by a sentence or two about innovation, the investigators, and the environment.

Keep your review succinct, bland, and businesslike: There will be many grants to review, so be succinct. If you are reviewer 2, you must not repeat what reviewer 1 just said. Briefly, highlight broad areas where you agree and disagree and focus your contribution on new points or nuances. Keep emotion out of the review. This is not a fight, it is not even a debate, it is a bland statement of opinion.

Disagree agreeably: If you disagree with another reviewer, there is no need to be aggressive. Usually something like, "I saw this somewhat differently," followed by your opinion is appropriate. If another reviewer is wrong, it is your responsibility to politely tell the group. For example, a reviewer might say, "They never included a sample size calculation." If you saw a sample size calculation, say so.

Don't nitpick: As a species, academics seem to enjoy pecking the intellectual offspring of their colleagues. We all have a tendency to want to show how smart we are by criticizing a piece of work. Remember, it is not possible for the applicant to include every detail or cover every eventuality in the grant. So be prepared to give applicants, particularly those who have proven they can address important questions successfully, some leeway. If in enthusiasm to show your intelligence and diligence, you nitpick and expose debatable weaknesses to the group, the best possible score for the grant with several minor weaknesses is 4.

After the meeting: You can edit your written on-line reviews after the meeting. You must edit your reviews if the wording is no longer concordant with your final impact score. You will also have to fill out a post-meeting conflict of interest. Destroy paper and electronic copies of the grants you reviewed and do not talk to anyone about the reviews. Add the grant review to your CV. The honorarium is automatically deposited in your bank account; you must declare it as income on your tax return; also, keep copies of your expenses because the *per diem* and ground travel allowance is taxable if you cannot show expenses.

Summary

1. Reviewing NIH grants is important for your career, accept the invitation.

2. Check your assigned grants early to make sure you don't have a conflict of interest.

3. Grant reviews are time consuming; allow enough time.

4. Your scores and text must be concordant.

5. Make a point of networking at the study section.

6. Don't nitpick to show how smart you are.

Resources

1. Information about the Early Career Reviewer program.
   https://public.csr.nih.gov/reviewerresources/becomeareviewer/ecr/pages/default.aspx

2. The NIH guidelines for grant reviewers.
   http://grants.nih.gov/grants/peer/reviewer_guidelines.htm

3. Videos about the NIH review process and study section.
   http://public.csr.nih.gov/ApplicantResources/Pages/default.aspx

Chapter 19

K to R and other career stress points

Why people do research?

It is hard to explain why some people enjoy research or are successful. You can list some of their characteristics: curious, persistent, accepting of risk, logical, creative, flexible, good writer, and so on. These do help, but they don't explain why someone does research. It is interesting that there are outstanding scientists in countries where research is poorly supported. What makes them do research in the face of such adversity? Some people are driven to pursue answers to questions by doing research no matter where they are. This drive, passion, or "fire in the belly" (mentor Grant Wilkinson), is something you need for success in research.

The trajectory of an academic research career

The Figure that follows illustrates a theoretical physician-scientist's career trajectory showing academic ranks and grants over time. It shows the idealized trajectory of someone who started research during the last two years of a clinical fellowship, was then supported by a training grant (T32 or F32) for three years, successfully applied for a K-career development award, and over five years transitioned to independence by obtaining an RO1 and then a second RO1.

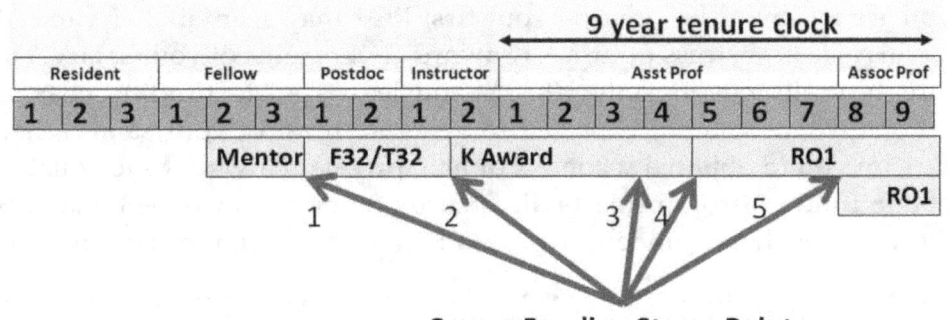

The Figure shows a hypothetical timeline for a physician-scientist. Each block filled with a number represents a year, and the blocks under them show the source of funding. Career stress points occur when progress depends on obtaining new funding and are shown by the arrows. A key to minimizing career stress points is to plan ahead – a key component of time management (Chapter 6).

The Figure illustrates several things. First, the process (even for this highly successful individual) is long. The average age at which investigators receive their first RO1 award is 42 for PhDs and 45 for MDs (1). Second, in addition to being long, the process also requires substantial training and mentoring and has several stress points where it is necessary to obtain funding in order to proceed.

Career stress points

1. The first stress point is the end of your first research year. Support for the first year of research is often easy – for example, research is usually a component of fellowship training. But this support is limited, if you wish to continue in research you will need funding from your mentor, or you will have to obtain funding through a T32 or F32 grant, or obtain a non-NIH grant.

2. The next stress point occurs at the end of a training grant. Training grants typically last two or three years; to continue research training, you will need a mentored career development award such as an NIH K-award, a VA CDA, or a faculty development award from a society (Chapter 11), or your mentor or institution will need to support you.

3. The end of your K-award is another stress point. K awards are a wonderful mechanism to train you to become an independent researcher. At the end of a K-award you will no longer be eligible for faculty development awards or K-equivalent awards, and you will need your own independent grant – usually an R award. The K-to-R conversion rate within five years of the K being awarded is 23% (19% in women and 25% in men), and after 10 years it is 43 % (36% in women and 46% in men) (2). In other words 6 out of 10 people who had a K-award did not get an RO1 within 10 years.

4. If you are a K-awardee, getting your first RO1 may seem like nirvana. Why should this also be a stress point? A K-award covers most of your salary, but an R-award typically covers only 30-50% and leaves a big funding chasm. At institutions where you are expected to generate most of your salary, there is pressure on you to obtain a second R or an equivalent award, or to collaborate and obtain funding from projects directed by other scientists. The majority of NIH RO1 holders have only one award (3); thus, collaboration is important.

5. At the end of your first R award there is stress related to renewing or replacing it. At many universities, if you are on the tenure track you have to fulfill the requirements for promotion to associate professor with tenure within a certain period of time – the tenure clock (Chapter 20). It is stressful to qualify for promotion within your tenure clock, and if your first RO1 finishes before you have applied for tenure, there is pressure to obtain another grant.

K to R

Congratulations! You got your K. Now what? A common mistake is to forget that the aim of a K is to get an R. The point of the K is to give you the training and opportunity to generate data for a successful R application, not to blindly pursue the original Aims of the K if common sense dictates otherwise. Once you have a K, you must set a timetable for your R application. For a 5-year K, your R needs to be submitted in year 3.5 or earlier. During your K, establish collaborations so that some of your effort will be on other people's grants when your K ends. During your K, discuss a strategy for the future with your mentor. You may need to meet with your head of department to discuss a "package" (Chapter 23).

Apply for lots of grants

To maintain funding, most successful researchers apply for more grants than they could ever accept because they know that most applications will not be funded. The worst that can happen is that if you are successful and overfunded you have to decline a grant. Concurrent grants may not provide support to do the same studies (termed "double-dipping"). Also, your percent effort cannot exceed 100%.

Percent effort

Your percent effort is based on all your professional work, including clinical work and work after office hours. It is not based on a certain number of hours. Let's say you are fully funded and working 60 hours a week and you get another grant that has 20% effort budgeted for you. You cannot say that you will increase your work hours by 20% to 72 hours a week and accept the grant. What you can do is reshuffle your effort on all your grants so that the total is less than 100%. Indeed, most institutions will not allow you to be 100% research funded because you would not be able to perform any non-research activities (e.g., teaching, committees). NIH can audit institutions (and thus individual investigators) to make sure that the effort they reported and charged to grants is true and related to research. Keep an eye on the effort you charge to particular grants to make sure that on average it reflects your activities related to the grant (including reading, writing, thinking, meeting, supervising, and performing the research).

You can adjust your effort if you need to. On most NIH grants, other than those that require a specified amount of effort, you can decrease effort by less than 25% without permission. So you can drop your effort from 20% to 16% without permission, but you need permission (approach your PO and have justifications ready) to decrease by 25% or more.

You cannot build stores for a rainy day

Unfortunately, unlike other competitive business models, you cannot build a reserve to protect against a rainy day. Most grants allow you to carry forward any unobligated balance into the next fiscal year. If you don't spend your year 1 budget, you can carry the surplus over into year 2. If the amount you expect to carry forward is more than 25% of the budget, you need to explain in your progress report why the funds accumulated and how they will be used. Also, if your entire funding period is completed and you have money left over in the budget you can request a one year no-cost extension (NCE). The first year of NCE is usually granted automatically, if there is still money left over after that year and the work is incomplete, you can apply for a second year of NCE.

Changing a career track is not failure

People can start on one track and switch to another. For example, if it becomes clear that a tenure-track career does not suit you, many institutions will allow you to change track a couple of years before your tenure clock runs out. Conversely, some people start on a clinician-scholar track but are so successful in their research and in obtaining grants that they change to the physician-scientist track. The teaching, patient care, and research endeavors of a large institution depend on many different skills and people. Finding a niche where you are happy, productive, and successful is not failure, it is success.

Have a Plan B

Funding for research has always fluctuated; a feast or famine Darwinian approach that makes little sense. Current (2018) pressures on scientists are particularly heavy. Many research-intense institutions expect scientists to stay fully funded at all times, but funding for research has decreased, the number of applications has increased, and paylines are tougher. Study sections cannot discriminate reliably between grants with the levels of precision demanded by single digit paylines (i.e., we cannot reliably distinguish between grants in the 9th and 15th percentiles). Because we cannot discriminate reliably between such grants based on their science, luck and academic politics play a greater role in funding outcomes. In addition to funding challenges, increased administrative requirements have made it more difficult to do research, particularly clinical research (4). Academic medical research is a wonderful career, but it is stressful and high-risk. Thus, in addition to keeping your sword as sharp as possible (Chapter 23), you must have a plan B in the back of your mind (i.e., what you would you do if, despite your best efforts, a research-intense career does not work out).

Summary

1. A career as an independently funded, tenure-track researcher has a trajectory with well-defined stress points.

3. The point of a K is to get an R.

4. Apply for an R in good time, keep your salary funded, and choose good collaborators.

4. One size does not fit all; there are many different successful career tracks and changing from one track to another often reflects success not failure.

Resources

1. NIH statements about new and early stage investigators.
http://grants.nih.gov/grants/new_investigators/index.htm
https://grants.nih.gov/policy/new_investigators/index.htm

2. Jagsi R, Motomura AR, Griffith KA, Rangarajan S, Ubel PA. Sex differences in attainment of independent funding by career development awardees. Ann Intern Med. 2009;151:804-11. PMID: 1994914

3. Pohlhaus JR, Jiang H, Wagner RM, Schaffer WT, Pinn VW. Sex differences in application, success, and funding rates for NIH extramural programs. Acad Med. 2011;86:759-67. PMID: 21512358.

4. Stein CM. Academic clinical research: Death by a thousand clicks. Science Translational Medicine 2015;7(318):318fs49. PMID: 26676604.

Chapter 20
Promotion and tenure

What is tenure?

The concept of academic tenure is in flux (1). Usually, tenure means that your position is guaranteed unless you are fired for serious misconduct. Historically, universities granted established professors tenure to provide them with academic freedom and to protect them from political or commercial pressure. In other words, someone with tenure could express opinions that might be unpopular without risk of being fired. Many academic medical schools have maintained university traditions, including the concept of tenure, but the meaning and worth of tenure at medical schools is often less well-defined than at universities.

What is tenure worth?

The worth of tenure is determined by what happens if you lose funding. If that happens, does tenure, in addition to guaranteeing your appointment, also guarantee your salary and job description? For example, if you have tenure and spend your time doing research, can your institution ask you to go back to seeing patients? Does tenure mean you keep an academic appointment and title but have no space or salary? It is difficult to find the answers to these questions because these policies are not always public. What we do know is that the answers differ among medical schools. A 2005 survey about tenure in 113 U.S. medical schools found that 38% of medical schools provided no financial guarantee, 9% did not clearly define a guarantee, 50% provided some financial guarantee, and only 5% guaranteed the total institutional salary (2). But even at schools where tenure has no financial worth, it has status value.

What is the tenure track?

The definition of tenure track varies, and some schools do not have a tenure track. If you are appointed on the tenure track it usually means the school recognizes that you want to focus your career on research and supports that plan. The tenure track identifies those scientists that an institution will invest in and ensure have protected research time (often contingent on the scientists generating salary). Some schools also include financial support such as a startup package with a tenure-track appointment, but many do not. The tenure track is designed to allow the best researchers to progress to a tenured appointment. Some institutions also have a tenure track for clinician-educators.

What is the tenure clock?

The tenure clock is the time during which you are expected to progress to a tenured position. The clock starts running when you are appointed on the tenure track (usually at the rank of assistant professor but sometimes instructor). After that, you have a fixed amount of time (usually between 7 and 9 years at different institutions) to meet the requirements for promotion from assistant to associate professor with tenure. This 7-9 year period is not just a trial period because many institutions have an "up-or-out" policy. In other words, if you do not make tenure you have to find another job. You can stop the tenure clock (temporarily) for having a child or serious illness. If you need to stop the clock, arrange this prospectively with the promotions committee through your department head. Don't wait until year 8 of a 9-year tenure clock to ask for time you missed in year 5 to be added retroactively.

What are the advantages of being on the tenure track?

You might reasonably ask why you should bother with this tenure-track time bomb if it doesn't seem to be worth much. Indeed, at some institutions there is little advantage to being on the tenure track; protected time for research is negotiated with your boss, and there is no "package" – resources depend on your success in research and obtaining funding, not on your track. Other institutions, however, provide support for tenure-track faculty. Also, some institutions are rigid and herd all potential career scientists into one track. Such an institution would not view you as someone committed to a research career if you are not on the tenure track. Additionally, some private funding bodies only consider people on the tenure track for their grants, but this requirement is falling away because some institutions no longer have a tenure track.

When to apply for promotion

At most institutions physician-scientists start at the rank of instructor and rise to assistant professor on the tenure track after it is clear they are committed and likely to succeed. Your promotion from assistant to associate professor is critical because that is usually when tenure is decided. You are ready for promotion when you unequivocally meet the research, funding, and stature criteria (described later). You must apply for promotion before your tenure clock runs out; at most institutions you have to start the application for promotion long in advance. For example, you might have to apply in year 8 if a decision about tenure has to be made before the end of your 9th year.

What if you are not ready for promotion and your tenure clock is running out?

If you are on the tenure track, you should monitor your progress and evaluate your chances of success towards the middle of your tenure clock. Discuss decisions with your mentor. If it seems unlikely that you will meet the criteria for tenure, you can usually request a change of track. For example, you could move from the physician-scientist track to the clinician-educator track. The rules for change of track vary. At some institutions you can apply for a change of track up to the end of year 5 of the tenure clock, others have less formal guidelines. If you decide to change track, don't view it as an admission of failure. People change tracks for many excellent reasons: fulfillment, family, a preference for clinical work, less stress, and a desire to develop more slowly.

Who decides if you should be promoted?

You will not be promoted automatically; someone (most often you or your division chief) has to initiate the process. A good division chief and mentor will keep track of your progress towards promotion, make suggestions along the way, and determine when you should apply. You too should track your progress and ask your mentoring committee for advice. If you, your mentor, and your mentoring committee feel you are ready for promotion, the first step is to meet with your division chief. Then, if you pass that hurdle, the division chief takes your case to the department chair and asks for support. If the chair supports your application, the process starts. The chair sends a letter of support and your promotion portfolio to the departmental promotion committee. This committee solicits opinions from external reviewers and decides whether or not to put your application forward to the next committee (usually the medical school promotion committee); that committee, if it agrees, passes your application on to the university promotion committee. The promotion process is time consuming and lengthy. The first step is preparing your portfolio.

Preparing your portfolio for promotion

Your institution will send you a list of what you need in your promotion portfolio. It usually includes documentation of your teaching contributions, a chair's recommendation letter, the names of 6-9 people who can provide an opinion about your research achievements, the names of 3-6 people who can attest to your teaching ability, and an up-to-date CV. Your CV must be impeccable (Chapter 21).

Referees for your research achievements

Most institutions require referees that are outside your home institution and that some be international. Generally, referees may not be your collaborators, people you have published with, or previous mentors. The rules vary, and sometimes there are time limits on the restrictions (e.g., you cannot use people as referees if you published with them in the previous five years).

Choosing your referees: Your referees should be from an institution comparable to yours (or better), and they should have a rank at least equal to the one you are applying for. You want to put forward the names of full professors at strong institutions. How do you come up with the names of 6-9 prominent people in your field? One way is to cultivate relationships with people who could be potential referees in the years leading up to your promotion. Make a point to meet visiting speakers and keep in touch with them at national meetings. Volunteer to serve on a committee for a national society. If you are on an NIH review panel, make a point of introducing yourself to the other members. Also, your mentor will have some contacts. Plan your list of referees in the years leading up to your application. The promotions committee, not you, sends the request for review to some of the individuals you have listed.

Criteria for promotion on the tenure track

Promotion on the physician-scientist and scientist tenure track at medical schools focuses on excellence in three areas – 1) scientific productivity, 2) funding, and 3) scientific reputation – and to a much lesser extent, contributions in other areas such as teaching, academic citizenship, and administration.

1) Scientific productivity: Reviewers judge the 1) quality, 2) number, and 3) trajectory of your publications. 1) Quality is hard to judge. Theoretically, reviewers should read all your papers and judge their quality. In reality, they judge based on a combination of the impact factor of the journals you published in and the number of times your papers have been cited. This makes it difficult for people in some subspecialties in which there are no high-impact (impact factor >10) journals and the research community is small. 2) The number of publications is easy to count. Promotion committees always say there in no magic number of papers that assures promotion; that is true, 10 papers in high-impact journals may be worth 50 in low-impact ones. Also, institutions and departments within an institution have different expectations. However, in a department of medicine at a good institution, approximately 30 or more original articles are the norm when people are promoted to associate professor (and 60 or more for promotion to full professor). 3) The trajectory of your publications shows whether you have been productive consistently, published in good journals, and been last author on some of your more recent publications.

> **H index:** An easy metric for a reviewer to obtain is your H-index (3). The H-index counts the number of papers that have been cited at least H times. If you have an H-index of 10, it means that 10 of your papers have been cited at least 10 times. It says nothing about the distribution of citations among those

10 papers. For example, five of those papers could have been cited hundreds of times. The H-index favors older established researchers because they have published more papers and there has been a longer time for others to cite them. The median H-index at promotion varies across institutions and scientific areas (e.g., neurosurgery vs. cell biology). An H-index of 10-15 and 20-30 are not unusual for promotion to associate and full professor, respectively. You can look up your H-index through *Web of Science* or *Google Scholar* (4).

Review articles: Review articles demonstrate scholarship but generally do not count much for promotion unless they are in high-impact journals. However, review articles are cited more frequently than original articles and can boost your H-index. As an early investigator, if more than 20% of your publications are reviews, it may suggest that your efforts are misdirected. Abstracts and letters to the editor do not count for promotion, and indeed can count against you if many abstracts never progress to papers.

First and last author papers: Reviewers are interested in your personal scientific contribution; they focus on first and last author papers to assess this. When you apply for promotion to associate professor you will need several last author papers to establish that you are scientifically independent. As a rule of thumb, you should be first or last author on a least half your papers. The letter from your chair, which your division director will draft (usually with your help), must highlight your scientific contributions and describe how they have advanced the field. The letter must allude to your work in the context of your career trajectory and future potential.

2) Funding: Promotion committees at different institutions use different criteria to evaluate how successful you have been in getting funding; at some you need to be the PI of an RO1 or equivalent, at others you need to have renewed an RO1, and at others you need more than just one RO1. The committees all want to know that you are likely to stay funded. A history of sustained success obtaining grants convinces them. The timing of your application in relation to your funding is important. Some people have struggled to get promoted after they had one or even two RO1s in the early years of their tenure clock but had no funding when they applied for promotion.

3) Scientific reputation: For promotion to the rank of associate professor you require a national reputation, and for full professor you require an international reputation. You can show the committee you have a national reputation with some of the following: serving on a committee for a national organization, serving on the program committee for a national meeting, giving invited talks at peer institutions in the US (even more impressive, internationally), serving on an NIH study section, serving on an editorial board for a good quality journal, reviewing papers for top tier journals, winning prizes, serving on advisory boards, and being recruited by another institution.

Other contributions: Promotion on the physician-scientist tenure track requires evidence of at least satisfactory performance in teaching, academic citizenship, and administration. Keep records of the classes you teach, the people you mentor, and any positive feedback or evaluation.

Criteria for promotion on the tenure track for physician-educators

Some institutions have a tenure track for physician-educators. Promotion on this track usually requires contributions to education that are nationally or internationally recognized and also solid research productivity and clinical work. The usual teaching we all do (even a lot of it) does not suffice. These individuals often develop and assess new ways to teach or evaluate the outcomes of education and direct courses or programs.

Criteria for promotion on the non-tenure track

Criteria for promotion to associate professor on the non-tenure track are not as strict as for the tenure track. The guidelines are similar, but fewer publications (approximately 20 or more for associate professor) are required, and there is no absolute requirement to obtain independent funding. Also, scientific productivity includes a broader range of scholarly activity so that review articles, book chapters, and middle author papers are viewed favorably. Documented excellence in teaching and clinical service is required.

Preparing for promotion

As your career develops, assess your academic progress in different areas against the criteria for promotion and adjust your activities accordingly. Use your mentor and mentoring committee to help you construct your portfolio and to identity and fix any weak areas.

Resources

1. Wald, C. Redefining tenure at medical schools.
   http://sciencecareers.sciencemag.org/career_magazine/previous_issues/art
   icles/2009_03_06/caredit.a0900032

2. Bunton SA, Mallon WT. The continued evolution of faculty appointment
   and tenure policies at U.S. medical schools. Acad Med. 2007 Mar;82(3):281-
   9. PMID: 17327718.

3. Carpenter CR, Cone DC, Sarli CC. Using publication metrics to highlight
   academic productivity and research impact. Acad Emerg Med. 2014
   Oct;21(10):1160-72. doi: 10.1111/acem.12482. PMID: 25308141.

4. Find your H-index. http://www.webofknowledge.com/

Chapter 21

Selling yourself – CVs, biosketches, and elevator speeches

Selling yourself

Part of being a successful scientist is to document your training, experience, work record, and achievements and to promote your work. You should prepare several major vehicles for selling yourself: 1) a long CV; 2) an NIH biosketch; 3) a one paragraph description of yourself; 4) an "elevator pitch"; and 5) a short resume (if you are applying for jobs in industry). You also need to keep track of your 6) conflicts of interest and 7) publications.

Accuracy is critical

Your CV represents you and your achievements. It precedes you to every job interview and scientific talk. Make sure everything in your CV and other biographic documents is absolutely accurate. Claiming degrees that you don't have, prizes you have not won, and experience you have not gained is dishonest and will get you fired or worse. Make sure there is no ambiguity. For example, if you claim a Rhodes scholarship, the reader will assume you mean the prestigious international scholarship to Oxford, not a scholarship from Rhodes, Iowa. Even though your Rhodes scholarship has the same name, you are misleading the reader. Or, if you say you worked somewhere from 2012 to 2013, the reader will assume it was a full time position. If it was not, make sure you say so. Details matter; one spelling mistake in a CV is a disaster.

1. Your long CV

Your CV should be neat, clear, concise, accurate, attractive, and easy to follow chronologically. A voluminous CV seems more impressive than a short one, but don't pad yours with marginally relevant information or use a creative layout to increase its length. As your career becomes more established, you can delete entries about minor achievements from your early career. For example, prizes and achievements at school are seldom relevant, and the importance of talks given to your own division wanes rapidly. Look at your mentor's CV and have your mentor look at yours. The layout of a long CV is fairly standard and most medical schools have a template they recommend. The Association of American Medical Colleges website (1) also has a template. Format your CV so that it is easy to follow chronologically and looks professional. There should be no unexplained chronological gaps – a reader should be able to work out where you were employed or studying at any time in the past. Number the pages. If you have nothing to record under a heading, leave the heading out. Photographs and personal information about age, date of birth, birth order, spouse, children, religion, hobbies, salary, and social security number are not required. Generally, the headings for sections of the CV are variations of those that follow and will be self-explanatory once you have looked at your mentor's CV.

Curriculum Vitae

Name
Work Address
Home-Address *Some people do not include a home address because if the CV finds its way onto the internet the information becomes public knowledge, others feel that this information is already public knowledge.*
Work Phone
Work email

Education
Postdoctoral Training
Certification and Licensures

Faculty Academic Appointments
Appointments at Hospitals/Affiliated Institutions
Other Professional Positions *Include advisory boards, committees, panels, and consultancies.*
Major Administrative Leadership Positions *Include courses and group activities you directed and committees you chaired.*

Committee Service
  Local
  National
  International

Professional Societies

Grant Review Activities *Include date, types of grant, and funding agency.*
Editorial Activities *Include any editorial board memberships and associate editor or editor positions; list journals you have reviewed for. Provides dates for board membership and editorial positions but dates are not required for reviews you performed for journals.*

Patents

Honors and Prizes

Grant Funding *Include grants on which you were the principal investigator and those on which you were a co-investigator, but make sure your status on the grant is clear – you don't want to give the false impression that all the grants are yours. Have subheadings that delineate current and past funding.*
  Current Funding
  Past Funding

Teaching
Invited Talks
  Local
  National
  International *Add other headings as appropriate for radio or television appearances.*

Publications *A common mistake on CVs is not to separate the publications into categories. Review articles and abstracts are considered less important than original research and reviewers like to have them separated.*
  Books
  Book chapters
  Reviews and Editorials
  Original Publications
  Abstracts and Letters

Trainees *Provide information about people you have mentored. You do not have to be the primary mentor in order to list a mentee; describe your mentoring role in a few words.*

Additional activities and skills *List activities that may be relevant (e.g., Experienced computer programmer proficient in R and SAS). Do not add mundane skills (e.g., proficient in Word and PowerPoint). I don't add information about hobbies but some people do.*

Your CV is a living document – groom and feed it regularly

The only way to ensure that your CV is complete, accurate, and current is to update it regularly. As soon as you publish a paper, give a talk, or win an award, add it to your CV. If you delay, you will either forget to add the information or you will make mistakes when you do. Include the PMID number for publications so that a reader can access the paper on PubMed. It is irritating when the PMID is incorrect – so download details about your publications into your CV through a reference manager or cut and paste the citation from PubMed (use the "Summary Text" format in "Display Settings" in PubMed) and then edit it. Only add unpublished papers to your CV after they have been accepted for publication and then provide the journal name followed by "In Press" or "Accepted for publication." Do not include papers that you have submitted for publication unless you are very early in your career and have few publications. Similarly, do not include papers that you are revising. If you decide to include papers you have submitted for publication, make sure 1) that the paper really has been submitted and you can provide a copy if requested, and 2) that the entry is current. It looks bad to see an entry for paper that was "submitted for publication" in 2015 on a CV in 2018.

2. Your NIH biosketch

You will need an NIH biosketch for every NIH grant application, and you can often also use it for non-NIH grant applications. The biosketch has a maximum length of 5 pages and a standard format – instructions, templates, and examples are available from NIH (2) and through links on the Association of American Medical Colleges website (1). The initial section of the biosketch includes your Name, Title, eRA Commons User Name, and Education/Training. This is followed by 4 sections: A. Personal Statement, B. Positions and Honors, C. Contribution to Science, and D. Research Support.

A. Personal Statement

The personal statement on your NIH biosketch should not be a generic paragraph that rehashes your CV. You should individualize at least part of it for the particular grant your biosketch is accompanying. Your personal statement needs to tell the reader not only what your qualifications are but also why you are particularly well-qualified to help answer the question this particular grant addresses. Some people write their personal statement in the first person (i.e., I am an Assistant Professor of…) others use the third person (i.e., Dr. Green is an Assistant Professor of…). Your personal statement should emphasize collaborations with other investigators on the grant, the skills and perspective you bring to the project, and your abilities to mentor, collaborate, or innovate, as appropriate. For example, for a K-award your personal statement would tell the reviewer about your past success in research, your relationship with your mentors, the training you already have, the training gaps you will fill, and your ability to collaborate and succeed. As a reviewer, I like it when K-applicants summarize their productivity: "I have published a total of 8 peer-reviewed original articles, 3 in the last year, including a paper in *Nature Communications*." In this section you can also, if need be, explain any reasons for gaps in your past productivity (e.g., illness, military service).

> **References after the personal statement:** You can reference up to 4 publications that highlight aspects of your personal statement. Not all investigators do so, perhaps because key references would be repeated in the "Contributions to Science" section. You are allowed to cite the same reference in different places; however, be careful because you don't want to seem to be milking a particular publication. I usually use the 4 references allowed after the personal statement to highlight papers showing collaboration with co-investigators on that grant. For example, in your personal statement for a career development grant you could write, "I have published six papers with my mentor and four are shown below."

B. Positions and Honors

List your previous positions in chronological order and conclude with your present position. List any honors such as prizes and awards. Generally, undergraduate awards are not relevant. If you have served on review or advisory committees, list them. You can also list membership of professional societies.

C. Contributions to Science

You are allowed to describe up to 5 of your most important contributions to science and to support each contribution with references to up to 4 of your peer-reviewed publications. I usually write this section in the first person. Your description of each of your contributions to science should identify the underlying problem and explain what you did or found that advanced the field. Each contribution should be no longer than about half a page (including the 4 references).

> **What if my contributions to science are small?** Reviewers do not expect scientists who are early in their careers to have 5 significant contributions to science each supported by 4 publications. One or two contributions with a couple of publications are fine. Also, remember that science is built on incremental advances; your work does not have to have won the Nobel prize for it to be a significant contribution. On the other hand, you don't want to inflate the importance of journeyman work. A bland scientific description of the work and why it was interesting is usually best. You should explain what your role in the work was if you are applying for a career-development award (e.g., I performed the NMR experiments, analyzed the data, and wrote the paper).

> **Have a heading for each contribution:** I like to have a heading for each scientific contribution and I tailor these according to the grant, even though the supporting references may be identical. For example, I have done work on the genetics of vascular response. If I am applying for a genetics grant, the heading for that contribution to science would be *Genetics of Vascular Response*, but for a non-genetics grant it would be *Regulation of Vascular Response*.

> **Which of your publications should you cite?** If you have a lot of publications, choose those that are more recent, have higher impact, and are related to the topic of the grant. If you have relatively few publications, you should usually include as many as possible within the framework of your Contributions to Science headings because reviewers of career development awards are looking for evidence that you are productive, energetic, and committed. However, you run the risk of appearing unfocused if your publications are in widely disparate areas. If that is the case, it may be wise to select those publications that tell the story of your current career path (and led to the grant application) or to use the personal statement section to subtly explain your unusual trajectory.

Example of a Contribution to Science section

C. Contribution to Science

1.<u>Oxidative stress in chronic HIV</u>

Improved therapy and survival in patients with HIV have led to the emergence of complications related to increased atherosclerosis. A possible cause is oxidative stress that can accelerate atherosclerosis by causing endothelial dysfunction. I tested the hypothesis that reducing oxidative stress in patients with HIV would improve endothelial function. I administered beetroot or placebo to patients with HIV and showed that beetroot improved both oxidative stress (F_2-isoprostanes) and endothelial function. I was responsible for all components of the study including design, recruitment, measurement of endothelial function (flow-mediated dilation), data analysis, and writing the paper. Based on our findings a larger trial is planned to examine the effects of improving oxidative stress on cardiovascular outcomes in patients with HIV. In additional studies using samples and data from this study, I showed that....

a. **Smith AA,** Jones BB, Brown CC. Improving oxidative stress in HIV-associated endothelial dysfunction. *HIV Res Proc* 2016;5:14-19. (PMC123456)....
b. Add publications b, c, and d.

Provide a link to all your publications: You also have the option of providing a URL to a full list of your publications in a publicly available database such as SciENcv or My Bibliography. Although you already maintain a CV and it is painful to create yet another list of publications, you should do so because reviewers do not have access to your full CV and cannot always judge your recent productivity from your biosketch. At the end of this chapter there are links to sites that will show you how to create the URL to your publications (3,4,5).

D. Research Support

If you have been supported by grants (i.e., part of your salary has been paid from a grant), list your current grants and (under a separate heading) those that were completed in the past three years. Include Federal and non-Federal grants. Provide the title of the grant, the principal investigator's name in parentheses, the funding agency, your role, and the dates of the grant. Do not include dollar amounts or your percent effort on the grant. You can also include a heading for "Pending Research Support" and list grants that you have submitted and are under review.

Example

D. Research Support

Current Support

1. Scientific Foundation Grant (Smith) 12/01/2016 – 11/30/2017
Scientific Foundation Research Starter Grant
This is a one-year grant designed to provide career development award funding.
Role: Principal Investigator

Previous Support
1. HIV Research Foundation (Jones) 07/01/2014-06/30/2015
High Innovation Award
The goal of this project was to understand the mechanisms underlying oxidative stress in patients with inflammation. Dr. Smith's role was to assist with subject recruitment.
Role: Co-investigator

Your biosketch must be flawless

Pay attention to detail; spelling mistakes or typos in your biosketch have a massive negative impact. Most investigators will be happy to share their NIH biosketches; examine several (particularly your mentor's) and have your mentor examine yours.

3. Your one paragraph description of yourself

A one paragraph description of yourself can be very helpful to colleagues who invite you to give a talk and have to introduce you. This paragraph usually highlights your past training, present positions, scientific achievements, honors, and anything else you particularly want the audience to know. An example follows.

Dr. Smith obtained her MD from the University of A in 1985. After a PhD under Dr Jones at University of B and a cardiology fellowship at the University of C she joined the faculty at the University of D in 1995 where she is Associate Professor of Cardiology and Director of the Heart Outcomes program. Her research focuses on understanding why patients with heart disease are not diagnosed and treated appropriately. She has published more than 50 papers in this area and has been elected to the Academy of Heart Failure Experts and awarded the Healthy Heart prize from the Cardiac Society.

4. Your elevator speech

You should have a brief (30 second) speech prepared for when you meet someone who asks, "So, what research do you do?" Treat the question as an invitation to "sell" your research and avoid the usual bland response, "Well, it's hard to explain, but I am working on lots of different things blah, blah." Rather, tell a story that gets the listener excited. Try the following format and practice out loud.

i) Define your broad area of passion: I am fascinated by discovering how to treat heart disease.

ii) Highlight a knowledge gap: There is a common heart rhythm problem called atrial fibrillation that we cannot treat very well.

iii) Pitch your hypothesis as a positive: We think that fish oil – something you could buy over-the-counter – may be an effective treatment for atrial fibrillation and we are testing it.

iv) Pitch the importance with a best-case scenario: If we are right, this could be a safe new treatment for atrial fibrillation that benefits millions of people.

You need different elevator speeches that are appropriate for lay-people, for scientists outside your area, and for aficionados. Similarly, if you meet the department chief in the elevator, have a positive, enthusiastic, one sentence answer ready for the usual small talk question, "How are things going?" The best answer is not, "So-so" or "Surviving," but something like, "Great. We have these fascinating preliminary findings showing that… and I am planning to turn it into an RO1 in the fall."

5. Your resume

Some people use the terms CV and resume interchangeably, so it can be confusing if someone asks for your resume. People referring to a resume in the academic context usually mean your long CV (although sometimes they are referring to your NIH biosketch). The term resume is used more often in the context of business. It contains many of the elements of the long CV but in a much more concise format and with a focus on achievements. A resume is usually between two and four pages long. A typical industry resume is two pages long, but in the healthcare industry a longer version, sometimes described as a hybrid between a CV and a resume, is often used.

Layout of the resume: The goal of your resume is to make you stand out from the pack. Just as with your CV, it should be attractive, accurate, and flawless. Avoid gimmicks like creative colors, photographs, artwork, and pithy aphorisms. Look at examples (6) and model yours accordingly. Resumes vary much more than CVs, but the usual headings are: Name with degrees, Contact Information, Executive Summary, Education, Experience, Awards and Honors, and Selected Publications. Some people begin their resumes (and CVs) with a heading "Objective" and write something like, *to achieve a fulfilling challenging position in the… industry that will allow me to…* The "Objective" heading is problematic because the usual objective is to get the job, and it is hard to say that in phrases that are original or inspiring. As a result, most people replace the "Objective" heading with an "Executive Summary" in the resume. Under this heading you summarize your major achievements and qualifications in few lines or bullet points.

Writing the resume: In contrast to the CV which is a bland, comprehensive, chronological list of your education and academic history, a resume highlights the story of your skills and achievements. Thus, resumes are rich in bullet points that list concrete achievements with action verbs that demonstrate leadership. For example, *Led the research group that developed the first assay for…; Co-inventor on two related patents; Designed* *and implemented a 2 credit hour class in molecular biology for a class of 30 undergraduates; Received the... award for excellence in teaching.* Resumes do have associated jargon, but phrases such as team-player, people-oriented, goal-oriented, problem-solver, and good communicator are hackneyed. It is preferable to illustrate the traits with concrete examples. Each job is different and it is worth tweaking the emphasis of each resume you send out so that it highlights your suitability for a particular job.

6. A conflict of interest log

If you have financial conflicts of interest (Chapter 27) or extra income it is useful to keep a running log. Some put in on their CV; I prefer to keep mine separate for my own use. If you have a log you don't have to rely on your memory when someone asks you to report conflicts of interest. I include dollar amounts so that I remember to report these earnings for my income tax. A log could look like this.

Cumulative conflict of interest/extra income log
2014 University of A: review of teaching program 2/23/2014 honorarium $1000
2015 ABC Pharmaceuticals: consulted on xy for hypertension 5/5/2015 $2500
         (Also re-imbursement of $825 travel expenses not taxable)
2016 NIH review: mail-in review 5/24/2016 honorarium $200

7. A file of all your publications

I keep a paper copy of all my publications, including abstracts. Some of my publications are in obscure journals that are not freely available and many of the abstracts are not available electronically. The file is helpful when I want to find information related to my own work, and it also inoculates me against someone accusing me of padding my CV with a non-existent publication or abstract.

Summary

1. Have an accurate, attractive, current, error-free CV.

2. Update your CV regularly.

3. Check your mentor's CV and have your mentor check yours.

4. Modify the text of your personal statement and scientific contributions on your NIH biosketch according to the grant you are applying for.

5. Prepare a 30 second elevator speech and practice it out loud.

6. Keep track of your conflicts of interest.

Resources

1. The Association of American Medical Colleges website has a template for a CV and provides useful guidance. https://www.aamc.org/members/gfa/faculty_vitae/150034/preparing_your_curriculum_vitae.html

2. Biosketch instructions, templates and examples. http://grants.nih.gov/grants/funding/424/index.htm#inst

3. To learn how to create a link to a list of your publications to My Bibliography. http://publicaccess.nih.gov/communications.htm

4. To add papers to My Bibliography through PubMed. http://publicaccess.nih.gov/my-bibliography-faq.htm#I.1.EnteringpublicationsintoMyBibliography

5. To generate the URL to share your bibliography. http://www.ncbi.nlm.nih.gov/books/NBK53595/#mybibliography.Sharing_My_Bibliography_a

6. Haseltine D. Job-search basics: how to convert a CV into a resume. Nat Immunol 2013;14:6-9. PMID: 23238749.

7. Grimes DA. Sabotaging your curriculum vitae. Obstet Gynecol 2010;115:1071-4. PMID: 20410784.

8. Some examples of CV's and resumes can be found at the following sites. http://www.resumagic.com/resume_sample_research_scientist.html http://career-advice.monster.com/resumes-cover-letters/resume-samples/sample-resume-research-scientist-midlevel/article.aspx

Chapter 22
Scientific meetings – schmoozing and posters

Meetings

Go to at least two meetings a year. One will be the big national meeting in your clinical area and the other a smaller subsection meeting. The national meeting will have thousands of attendees; however, people with similar interests cluster at particular study groups or poster sessions. When you go to a meeting you should plan carefully. The point of going to a meeting is to showcase your work and to meet people. To meet people you have to talk to people, even if this is not something that comes to you naturally. Before you go to the meeting, make a mental list of a few leaders and potential collaborators in your area who will be there and research their work on PubMed. At the meeting, talk to as many of them as possible. Remember, the goal of networking is not shake hands with as many people as possible; it is to develop and keep a few key contacts. (But to do that you do have to shake a lot of hands.) People may not remember you after one meeting, but after they have seen you a few times they recognize you and your work. All this takes effort on your part. If there are leaders or collaborators that are particularly important to you, ask your division chief to invite them to your institution to give a talk. When that happens, spend time with them and then make a point of looking them up at the next meeting.

Connect with your peers: Perhaps even more important than connecting with a couple of influential people is connecting with your peers. Make an effort to connect with people at your level and exchange war stories; they are your future friends, collaborators, and reviewers. You want them to know you are a good scientist, collaborator, and colleague. Over the years, the more times you connect with the same people the stronger your relationships with them.

Go to smaller meetings: The smaller subsection meeting will usually have less than a thousand attendees and its focus should be much closer to your research area. Look for the same people you met at the big national meeting – greet them by name, go to their posters and talks, and if they come to your posters, chat with them. Some mentors recommend that you ask a question at every talk you attend. I think this is silly. The audience soon recognizes you and your strategy and groans inwardly every time you stand up to ask a question.

Prepare for the meeting: Big meetings are chaotic. There are thousands of people milling around trying to find meeting rooms. You cannot just arrive and plan to wander around to see what you find interesting. Before you go to the meeting, work your way through the on-line program and plan each day. Also, work your way through the abstracts by searching on key words relevant to your areas of interest (or relevant to the people you want to meet). From your search write down (or use the meeting app) the abstracts that interest you. For posters, I have a hierarchy. On each day I flag 4 or 5 posters that interest me so much that I want to meet the presenters, then I list the other posters I want to see. I visit my important posters first because once I start going around the posters it always takes longer than I expected.

Don't let meetings depress you: It is easy to become envious (Chapter 28) and feel inferior when you see the wonderful work your brilliant competitors have done. Program your mind to absorb and process ideas without comparing and judging. If you lapse into comparisons, remind yourself of your own wonderful achievements. After the meeting, reflect on what you have learnt and adjust your research priorities if need be.

Posters

Poster presentations are a great vehicle to make you more visible and connect with other scientists at meetings.

Making a poster: Your poster should be attractive, legible from a minimum of six feet away, and informative. I don't believe in spending a lot of time making posters, so my format and color scheme (black text, white background) are simple, and I use the same text as in the abstract. I know this text is accurate and error free; I cut and paste relevant parts of it into the different sections of the poster as bullet points and enlarge the font so that is is easily legible. I then add data tables and figures to make the poster attractive and more informative than the abstract. There are excellent online guides on how to make a poster (1). PowerPoint is convenient (2); it is easiest to use someone's existing PowerPoint poster as a template and modify it. The biggest mistake novices make is to cut and paste text from the draft of a paper into the poster. This results in dense illegible text and a horrible poster (3). People who chat to you at your poster do so because they are either good-natured chatty souls or interested in the topic. Both groups will chat to you provided your poster is legible.

Getting your poster there: Double-check that there are no spelling errors in the title. Then roll the poster up and carry it with you so that if your luggage is lost you still have your poster. Also carry an electronic copy of the poster on a thumb drive so that in an emergency you could print another poster. Most meetings provide poster pins, but it is prudent to take some of your own. Arrive in good time to mount your poster. Later, remove it at the appointed time because the organizers often discard posters that have not been removed in good time.

You cannot present a poster if you are not present: Meetings display posters at a certain time (e.g., 8-10 a.m.) and ask poster presenters to be present for part of that time (e.g., 8-9 a.m.). You should be present during your allocated time, because if someone particularly wants to meet you, this is when they will visit. If you have more than one poster on display during your allocated time, you can leave a note on one poster directing traffic to the other where you are in attendance.

Presenting a poster: There are different poster presentation styles. Every poster presenter feels awkward when people glance at the poster title for a second and pass by, assiduously avoiding eye contact. As a result, some poster presenters get a hangdog look, and others insulate themselves from rejection by sitting on a chair and reading. It is important to have a positive and confident presence. At the same time, you do not need to accost everyone who glances at your poster. If someone stops at your poster and is reading it, you can say something like: "Let me know if I can explain anything," or "Would you like me to walk you through it?" If someone asks you to explain the poster, it is safe to start with the short version lasting about a minute with about 5 sentences: "We were interested in x because y; We randomized two groups (pointing to Table 1) to b and c and measured d; We found xy (pointing to Figures); We think this is important because…; I have given you the very short version and would be delighted to expand." Activity at a poster draws activity. Introduce yourself to poster presenters around you; look at their posters and show them yours. Don't let an old friend monopolize your attention with social chit chat; if you are talking to someone and another person is obviously waiting to ask a question, you should bring that person into the conversation: "Did you also have a question?" Make sure you have business cards and that your email address is on the poster.

Resources

1. Practical guidance on making a poster. http://guides.nyu.edu/posters

2. How to make poster in PowerPoint.
   http://undergraduateresearch.as.ua.edu/presenting-your-work/making-posters/

3. Erren TC, Bourne PE. Ten simple rules for a good poster presentation. PLoS Comput Biol. 2007 May;3(5):e102. PMID: 17530921

Chapter 23

Getting your next job – keeping your sword sharp

Why do people move?

Academic scientists change institutions relatively frequently, usually for a combination of reasons that push or pull. Common pushes are lack of support (mentoring, research resources, money, and collaborators), difficulty differentiating from a mentor, feeling undervalued by leaders, and a partner moving. Common pulls to new institutions are a promotion, a leadership position, a title, more money (salary or support for a research program), more protected time, better resources and collaborators, and job security (i.e., some guaranteed salary support).

Moving can be dangerous for early career investigators

In Chapter 4 I discussed why moving for the wrong reasons is dangerous. Leaving an established mentor and an environment that made you successful is a major step. You shouldn't move just because of a fancier title, a bigger office, or a higher salary. You should only move if the new environment is much better for your research and you can collaborate with a great mentor at the new institution.

Keep your sword sharp even if you don't intend to move

You are responsible for your career. Even if you are not looking for a new position, it is important to stay marketable – it is you best job security (1). Your worth in an academic environment is ephemeral and there is a strong "what have you done for me today" mentality. Institutions act in their own best interests and have no loyalty to individuals. You cannot foresee an institution's future commitment to you when times get tough. I liken the careers of academic scientists to those of warriors: we fight loyally for a group and a leader, but if the situation changes we take our swords and join a new group. To remain marketable you must have funding, productivity, visibility, and connections with leaders.

Becoming and staying visible

When you start as a scientist, you are invisible to the scientific world. You become visible in a research area in the following ways: 1) publish great papers;

2) go to meetings and present data; 3) give invited talks; 4) write reviews; 5) serve on committees and study sections; and 6) collaborate with other researchers. You can see why it is important to focus your research – it is difficult to become visible and establish a reputation in even one area. Remember too, you must have a national and international reputation (manifestations of visibility) to meet the criteria for promotion and tenure.

1) Publishing: Publications, both their number and quality, are key to your visibility and success. Aim at journals that increase your visibility.

2) Meetings: Go to at least two meetings a year and use them to promote yourself effectively (Chapter 22).

3) Invited talks: Generally, if someone invites you to give a talk, you should accept and use the opportunity to meet as many people as possible.

4) Review articles: Promotion committees do not "count" review articles as scientific publications towards promotion on the physician-scientist track. Therefore, you should be selective about the number and type of review articles you write because they take time away from your research. However, review articles in journals that are high-impact or that your research colleagues esteem make you more visible and enhance your reputation in an area.

5) Serving on committees and study sections: Committees can be a time sump, but committees outside your institution are great networking opportunities. If you serve on an NIH study section, your reputation grows and you can network with a new group. Make a point of introducing yourself and chatting with key people at committee and study section meetings. These people can be excellent future external referees when you apply for promotion (Chapter 20).

6) Collaborating: If you collaborate with leaders or future leaders, you will not only improve your science but also your visibility. It is better to collaborate with people than to compete with them.

Getting your next job

Scientists move either because someone approached them out of the blue about a position, or they actively sought a new job.

Not actively looking: Even if you are not actively looking for a job, someone may contact you and ask if you are interested in a position. If you say yes, you trigger a cascade of events, discussed later. If you say no, you close a door. If you are happy and successful, and the enquiry is from an institution that is not a step up for your science, you should not waste everyone's time. But if the enquiry is from an institution you are interested in, there is no harm in finding out about the position. Remember, the "recruitment package" is ephemeral (Chapter 4) and you must base your interest on the wellbeing of your long-term research career.

Actively looking: How do you look for a new academic job? There are three common approaches: 1) checking advertisements; 2) contacting academic divisions; and 3) networking. All three are important. Major journals such as *NEJM, JAMA* and *Nature* advertise jobs. If you apply, follow the instructions and make sure your cover letter is appropriately formal and without errors. However, many jobs are not advertised. It is fine to send an unsolicited email of enquiry to a division chief at an institution that interests you. Your email should be formal, beginning *Dear Dr. Jones* and ending *Sincerely, Ann Smith*, and you must attach your CV. Make sure the email you send is not generic, e.g., *Dear Division Director, I am interested in a career as a physician-scientist at your institution...* Address your email to a particular person at a particular institution, describe your background and aspirations briefly, and say what you think you can contribute to the division (to do that you need to know what is going on in the division). To network for jobs ask your mentors to activate their networks and activate your own. Contact your colleagues and friends, and if you have given talks at other institutions, let the people there know you are looking for a new position.

The pro's and con's of looking at other jobs: Even if you are not actively looking for a new job, there are several advantages to looking at some of the positions people contact you about. First, you may find your dream job. Second, you learn about different institutions and their academic workings. Third, you meet senior scientists who think you are good enough to recruit, and even if you don't take their job, they can be great referees when you later apply for promotion. Fourth, efforts to recruit you validate your value in the marketplace, and your institution might review your current package. Not unexpectedly, packages for outside recruits tend to be more generous than the support offered to home-grown individuals.

There are also disadvantages to looking at new positions. First, if word gets around that you are interviewing elsewhere, it can lower morale in your laboratory. Second, the leadership at your home institution might decide that you are not worth investing in because you clearly want to leave. This is particularly a risk if you recently negotiated a better package with your institution after you had an offer from elsewhere, and here you are looking at yet another job.

Interviewing

Once someone expresses interest in you, the interview dance has predictable steps: preamble, preparation, a talk, interviews, dinner, the end of the visit, a second visit, negotiating, a go or no-go decision, and moving (or staying).

Preamble to the interview: There is usually a preliminary phone call to discuss your level of interest and general suitability for the position and to decide if you should be invited for an interview. If someone has called you out of the blue, it is fine to say something like: "I am happy where I am and not actively looking, but the position sounds interesting and I would be delighted to look at it." This can elicit the response, "What would it take for you to move?" Prepare a suitable answer that deals with generalities not specifics, and remember the best answer has nothing to do with money; it is about how you can contribute to the success of the institution and how your program can flourish. After this preliminary conversation you might be invited to visit.

Preparation for the visit: You should prepare for your visit. Research the institution and division that you are visiting. Ask to meet with particular people that are potential collaborators. When you receive the agenda for your visit, research each person on your schedule and prepare some questions. Dress appropriately; it is better to be a little overdressed than underdressed. Pay attention to your appearance and the image you project. Your shoes should be clean and good quality, your clothes should be businesslike but not flashy, keep jewelry and perfume or aftershave to a minimum, don't smoke, and don't chew gum. Have some knowledge about the city you are visiting.

An interview talk: You will be asked to present a talk. Prepare and rehearse an outstanding talk that is appropriate for your audience (Chapter 24). Make sure you are aware of and refer to relevant work from the local institution and mention any existing collaborations you have with local faculty.

Interviews: You will spend most of your time moving from person to person for a series of interviews. This is exhausting. Prepare a brief description of yourself in response to the frequent question: "Can you tell me a bit about yourself?" Prepare answers for other obvious questions (e.g., "Why are you looking for a position? What about us interests you? What will you need to be successful? How do you see yourself fitting in here? Where do you see yourself in five years?"). Your answers shouldn't be too long but designed to keep a two-way conversation going. Be positive about yourself, the world, your current institution, and the future. This is not the place to complain or vent. Have some questions ready for each interview. If someone asks uncomfortable questions about your specific needs, you can deflect them at this stage by asking about what is usually provided by the institution for new recruits. For example, you may be asked, "What (salary, lab space, package) are you looking for?" A reasonable (and fact-gathering) response would be, "I will have better idea of that after my visit, but can you tell me what the usual approach here is to (salary, lab space, package) for new recruits."

Dinner: The interview process does not end with the interviews. You will be evaluated all the time, by everyone you meet – drivers, secretaries, students, and professors. At dinner be punctual, polite, pleasant, positive, and conversational. Do not have more than one alcoholic drink.

The end of the visit: At the end of the visit you will meet with the person who invited you and discuss how the visit went. The questions will assess your level of interest and identify areas that could be obstacles to you moving. At this stage, there will usually not be concrete negotiations; the meeting is to discuss whether you wish to proceed with the process and what the next steps will be. Within a few days of arriving home, send a brief email or handwritten note to all the people you met thanking them for meeting with you. Your contact person will be in touch once the interviewing team has met all the candidates and synthesized their opinions. If you never hear back, you can assume they were not interested in you and there is not much point in enquiring further.

When and how to tell your home institution: It is helpful to involve your mentor every step along the way even though you might find it awkward to tell your mentor you are looking at a job. Much more awkward is deciding what to tell your division chief. The temptation is to say nothing. I don't think this is the best approach, although it is what I did. (I felt that if I wanted to move I would, and if my home institution suddenly expressed greater interest in me, this was a response extracted under duress and would not factor into my decision.) News that you are interviewing elsewhere can leak at any time and ring alarm bells in your home institution, so rather than wait for the information to leak, it is courteous to tell your division chief. Some advise you to do this immediately after the first visit; others suggest you only do it if you plan a second visit. Because the first visit is a bilateral look-see without any commitment, I think it is reasonable to say nothing about the visit if you have no intention of proceeding. If news leaks and someone asks, you can reply, "Yes, they asked me to visit and I did but I wasn't interested in pursuing it." You should tell your division chief if you return for a second visit and also if you receive an offer letter. Although you want to inform your chief, you don't want to come across as someone playing the game to get a better deal. A reasonable way to approach it is: "I didn't want you to be blindsided so I want to let you know that University of X has asked me to interview." This will usually stimulate questions about your initial thoughts and how far things have progressed. Be positive about both institutions; this is not the time (in fact, no time is appropriate) to be critical of your home institution and the support you have received.

The home institution's response: Your home institution can respond to the news that you are interviewing in several ways: 1) silence; 2) suggest the move will be good for you (and please close the door on the way out); 3) say that you are highly valued but nothing more can be offered; 4) offer to start discussing what you need; 5) ask to discuss matters when you receive an offer. Be prepared for any of these responses and don't let them cloud your decision. Separate fact from emotion.

Pride and punishment: One common emotion that should not drive your decision is pride (i.e., you feel obliged to leave because you told your department head you were looking elsewhere and no-one did anything about it – suggesting to you that you are not valued). Another common emotion is to want to leave to "punish" an institution that has not valued you highly enough. I think we all feel this emotion because institutions are impersonal and do not communicate appreciation well. They do, however, communicate inequality well; there will always be people who (in our eyes) were treated better in terms of space, titles, money, accolades, and support. The niggling possibility that we have been chronically undervalued suddenly flares when an outside offer validates our estimated self-worth and gives rise to an irrational desire for "revenge." Don't get sucked in by these emotions. Your future scientific success is the critically important variable in your decision, not whether you feel valued. Ask your mentor for advice.

A second visit: If someone contacts you after the first interview, it will be to talk about the next steps. If they like you and you like them, the negotiations could proceed rapidly by telephone and email. If they are uncertain, or you are uncertain, or if you will fill an important position and cost them money, they could invite you back for a second visit. A second visit is much like the first except there is more emphasis on logistics and you are often not asked to give another talk. You might get to look at your potential laboratory space, core service laboratories, schools for your children, and places to live. Also, if you have a partner, both of you might be invited to visit. If you are invited for a second visit, you should assume they are seriously interested in you, and you should not go unless you are interested enough in them in them to want more information.

Negotiating: A negotiation is not an argument nor is it mainly about you; it is a fact-finding conversation that will result in an agreed plan that benefits both parties. The process is less about the person and more about the mission (Josh Fessel). It is not about them giving as little as possible and you getting as much as possible; it is about common interests – you must understand and explain how the outcome of the negotiation serves both their interests and yours.

There are many excellent books on negotiation and you should read a couple. The key themes in these books are: 1) know your facts; 2) know what you want; 3) listen to the other side's point of view and understand their needs; 4) explain why your point of view is good for them; and 5) have some flexibility. There are two main reasons to negotiate: the first and most important is to ensure that you have everything you need to be successful and that there are no surprises; the second is that the best time to ask for things is when you are being recruited. Studies suggest that women are less likely to negotiate than men, and that this may account, in part, for the salary differential between men and women that persists even in later years at some institutions.

Negotiating: 1) Know your facts Before you start negotiating, it is important to understand how a particular institution works. Research their policies and benefits on-line, speak to contacts who know that system, and during your interviews gather information about what a possible offer might look like by asking about the "usual" processes regarding career tracks, clinical load, teaching load, protected time, promotion, tenure, support for a new recruit, space, etc. Many public universities publish their salary scales. Keep your relative "strength" in mind. Are you negotiating from a position of strength (e.g., fully funded for the next 5 years) or from a position of relative weakness (e.g., you are in the last year of a K-award and your RO1 application was not scored)?

Negotiating: 2) Know what you need, want, and dream Negotiators sometimes talk about knowing your "walk-away" number (the absolute minimum you would accept). This is a number that you do not share with the other side, but it provides a floor for your negotiating. The same concept applies to academic negotiations – make a list of what you absolutely must have to be successful and make sure that the offer you accept provides at least this. This list is almost like a business plan: it should include essential people, space, equipment, lab supplies, animals, animal care facilities, research nurses, and so on with estimated costs for each item except space (unless the institution charges for space). Think about needs beyond science (e.g., you might have a partner that will also relocate and need a suitable position). In addition to making sure you have what you need, you can ask for things you want, but make sure you can justify your requests in terms of mutual success. If you dream about unusual resources, find out what the institution's dream is for your area – if your two sets of dreams are concordant, you may be able to push for support to realize your mutual dream.

Negotiating: 3) Know what they need, want, and dream An institutional negotiator wants you, and therefore the institution, to be successful. You must understand why you are being recruited. What need does the institution want you to fill? If you understand their perspective and frame your conversation about your needs and requests in the light of how they will help you fulfill the institution's needs (minimum), wants (desires), and dreams (shoot for the stars), you are more likely to get what you want.

Negotiating: 4) Explain why your point of view is good for them You should always be positive, cordial, and diplomatic, and you must have facts to back up your requests. The person you are negotiating with may not understand anything about your science; thus, you have to explain what you need to be successful and why each thing you ask for is important. The point is not to "get as much out of them as possible" but to get what you need to be successful and thus make them successful – in other words, this is a collaboration not a battle.

Negotiating: 5) Have some flexibility Remember that the negotiator has limited space, money, and flexibility and is sensitive to precedents in the institution. If you are offered a deal that is much better than what someone of similar rank in the same division received, it will lead to internal discord. Negotiations work best if there is some give-and-take; do not expect to "win" every point you negotiate. Decide which points are really important and be prepared to "give" on some of the less critical ones.

Negotiating: The offer letter If an institution is interested, there will be an offer, or talk about what an offer might look like, as a way of opening serious negotiations. The offer letter will cover items 1-5 that follow. Once you are no longer talking generally but negotiating specific details in the offer, you are implying that you are ready to move and it it just a question of sorting out the details. So if you have already decided you're not interested in moving, it is not worth going further just to see what their best offer might be. Some people, however, do continue negotiating and use the final offer letter as a tool to obtain a better deal at their home institutions. If there is no formal offer letter and only a verbal agreement, it can be helpful to summarize the conversations regarding items 1-5 in an email. For example, "It was great talking to you and I am very excited by the opportunity. To make sure I understood our conversations correctly I tried to summarize them. I will be appointed at the rank of… My salary will be… and my lab will…" Therefore, it is important to make notes of important conversations. Alternatively, you can ask the person you spoke with to summarize the areas covered; I prefer to do it myself because then I control the wording. Beware of future promises: "We don't have a lab on campus for you right now, but the space downtown is only three miles away and you will be on the top of the list for the new building."

At many institutions the offer letters for instructor and assistant professor positions are generic, and there is not much room for negotiation unless you are an unusually desirable candidate (your research into the institution should already have told you which areas are negotiable). The offer covers the following areas: 1) title and track; 2) clinical duties; 3) salary; 4) generating your salary; and 5) space and resources. The support offered is sometimes called a recruitment package and is not related to the benefits package (retirement, health insurance, disability insurance) which is usually fixed. However, it is very important for you to find out exactly what benefits are offered and to read the fine print. For example, if your disability insurance does not kick in until you have worked for a year you might need to take out additional insurance.

1) *Title and track:* Your title will usually be obvious: Instructor or Assistant Professor in the Division of… in the Department of… A big question is your track. At some institutions the instructor rank does not count towards the tenure clock. If this is the case, you might want to start as an instructor if your research career is undeveloped. On the other hand, if you already have several publications and independent grant support, you might ask for the rank of assistant professor. Irrespective of rank, everyone (including you) needs to understand what track you will be on, because different tracks carry different expectations and criteria for evaluation (Chapter 1).

2) *Clinical duties:* The biggest determinant of your protected research time will be your clinical duties. Your clinical commitments must be specified ahead of time and the division chief must agree with the proposal. Protected time is key to the success of physician-scientists, and many institutions limit the clinical load to approximately a half-day clinic a week and one month a year attending on the wards. Define what other duties you will be expected to perform (e.g., teaching, academic service, committees, resident supervision).

3) *Salary:* When you start looking for a job, get an idea of the salary range for a position like yours. Research the Association of American Medical Colleges (AAMC) report on medical school faculty salaries and speak to your peers and mentors. Most academic medical center libraries have the AAMC report or can provide you electronic access to it. Your salary is generally set by local institutional guidelines and there may be little flexibility. It is also the least important component of your success. However, your future salary will track based on its starting point, so make sure the starting point is reasonable.

4) *Generating your salary:* A key question is how you will generate your salary. If you have grant funding that covers your entire salary, you are a bargain for any institution. However, many early researchers arrive with a K-award or a single RO1 that does not cover their entire salary. An institution that wants to hire you will recognize this and guarantee your salary for a number of years to give you time to establish your research and get additional grant support. A proposed recruitment strategy of: *If you don't get that RO1 you just submitted, we can always arrange for you to do a few extra clinics until you get a big grant,* is a recipe for failure. Protected research time is even more important after you move than at other times. Your protected time will not last forever, and unless you obtain grants to support your research, you can expect to increase your clinical load once the protected time guaranteed in your recruitment package expires.

5) *Space and resources:* You should be given an office, a computer, and laboratory space, and you might be given money to support part of a technician or nurse as part of your package. Sometimes an institution will provide a lump sum of "development funds" that you can use to hire someone or buy equipment. If there is a lump sum, check whether it expires after a certain time or if you can keep it for a rainy day if you do not use it immediately. It is important for the institution that you are successful. Therefore, it is important for you to ask for the resources you need to be successful. If there is key equipment you need, make sure you have access to it, that the equipment works, and that it can accommodate an extra user. Make sure your laboratory space can handle the experiments you will do and is located with reasonable access to large equipment you will use. Find out what administrative support there is for tasks such as grant applications, scheduling appointments, and booking travel. If you have identified a local mentor, you can ask for guidance.

Negotiating: After the offer letter Once you have received the offer letter, don't decide immediately. You should, however, respond immediately. Acknowledge receipt of the letter and say when you will get back to them, Dear Dr..., Thank you very much for your offer letter which I received. I am honored by this exciting opportunity. Can I ask for two weeks to think about this... Unless you definitely want to leave your home institution (and probably even then) it is good form to tell your division chief about the offer letter. If you would like to stay at your home institution provided it comes up with a good deal for you, it is reasonable (if asked) to share the offer letter you received with your division chief. But after that, trading subsequent offer letters between the competing parties to see who will bid the highest is crass.

Evaluate your choices with your mentor and plan a strategy. Some people find it helpful to make a list that compares institutions. The list will have things like research support, collaborators, mentors, resources, reputation, protected time, and so on. You can allocate each item on the list a weight (e.g., resources=30% of my decision) and then score each institution. So for resources University A might be stronger and score 20/30% and University B scores 15/30%. Then you sum all the scores for A and B and see which has the better score. Although it does force you to compare institutions side-by-side, I don't think this system works very well because most people make difficult decisions based on their gut not their head. If you are debating, remember that a move should improve your situation substantially, not just a little. In fact, some say that you should only move if the improvement in resources and opportunity is 50% or more (1). So, if you are debating there is probably no debate.

If you are serious about moving, think about whether you need to negotiate aspects of the offer letter. If so, make a list in order of importance, because if there are 5 points on your list you might only get some "give" on the first few. Respond with positive energy before you ask for anything (e.g., *I am excited by your letter and believe University of X would be a great fit for me and that I would contribute etc. I wanted to ask if we could discuss a few points in the offer letter*).

Be prepared for the recruiting team to ask you about a potential counteroffer from your home institution and whether you would be willing to share it with them so that they could match components of it. I think it is reasonable to say that you'd be happy to discuss aspects of a counteroffer, but I don't think trading offer letters back and forth is a good idea. Remember, this negotiation is about your success (and the institution's) and not about getting as much as you can.

Moving: Moving is stressful. Most institutions cover some of your moving expenses; use that resource to minimize your stress. Unless there is a good reason not to do so, tell your mentor about the new job as it develops and seek advice. You will need to discuss how to complete your current experiments, future collaborations, and how to be successful at your new institution. It can take many months for you to get a medical license in a new state and credentials at a new hospital – start the process early. Ideally, you should have those documents in hand before you move.

Resources

1. Simone JV. Understanding academic medical centers: Simone's maxims. Clin Cancer Res 1999;5:2281-5. PMID:10499593

2. Office of Career and Professional Development, University of California, San Francisco. Negotiating your start up package. https://www.google.com/?gws_rd=ssl#q=%22negotiating+your+startup+package

3. Boss JM, Eckert SH. Academic scientists at work: negotiating a faculty position. http://www.sciencemag.org/careers/2005/02/academic-scientists-work-negotiating-faculty-position-0

4. Fisher, R., Ury, W. and Patton, B. (1991). Getting to Yes: Negotiating Agreement Without Giving In. Second Edition. New York: Penguin Books.

Chapter 24
How not to give a bad talk

You may not be a born orator but that is no excuse for giving a bad talk

How many times haven't you sat through a talk wishing the miserable hour would end quickly? This is entirely the fault of the speaker, because you came to the talk interested and wanting to learn about the topic. The speaker failed to provide the goods. Worse, the speaker tortured you. Most of us will never be wonderful orators and captivate an audience. However, there is no excuse for giving a bad talk. To avoid giving a bad talk you need to think about six areas: 1) the invitation; 2) preparing the content; 3) preparing the slides; 4) preparing the delivery; 5) the delivery; and 6) the postmortem.

1. The invitation

At some time in your career you will receive an email, *Dear Dr. Smith, Congratulations, your abstract has been selected for an oral presentation at the National Meeting of...*, or a colleague will invite you to give a talk about your work, or someone will invite you to give medicine grand rounds, or you will give a talk as part of a job interview. These are different types of talks and require different preparation; however, the same general principles apply to all. My first response to the invitation is usually panic and to think of all the reasons why it is impossible to do the talk: I don't have anything to talk about, I don't have time to prepare the talk, I'd have to leave my family for two days….and so on. Whether you accept or not should be influenced by the type of invitation.

There are different kinds of invitations: You will receive many spam email invitations to give talks at meetings you've never heard of, with people you've never heard of, about topics that seem barely related to your work, and to pay your own way. These meetings are moneymaking rackets and are not worth attending.

If your work is related to a drug, you might be invited to talk at a meeting sponsored by a company. There is nothing wrong with speaking at such meetings, provided that there is no direct or indirect influence on what you say and that the meeting is for scientific and not marketing purposes (Chapter 27). Reject meetings that provide you with prepared slides, or that want to pre-approve the content of your slides. Also, beware of meetings that do not pass the smell test – for example, an all-expenses-paid weekend for you and a partner at a ski resort for giving a 30 minute talk. Most invitations to speak will be legitimate and will come from institutions or organizations that you know. You should accept these invitations.

Say yes to the invitation: Until you are tenured or have given many invited talks outside your institution, accept all (or as many as possible) invitations. There are many reasons to do this. 1) One of the criteria for promotion on both the physician-scientist and clinician-educator tracks is your national and international reputation. One of the ways you build your reputation is to give invited talks. International talks are considered particularly prestigious. 2) A talk gives you an opportunity to highlight your work and its importance. 3) You have the opportunity to promote yourself within the circle of people who will review your grants and papers and will be recommending candidates to search committees for future jobs. 4) You will meet people interested in your work and this can lead to new collaborations and ideas. 5) The preparation for a talk forces you to review the recent literature and think critically about your work.

Solicit invitations to talk: If you're not getting invitations to talk, discuss this with your mentor who may be turning down invitations and could pass them on to you. Also, there is nothing wrong with tactfully prodding your network or your mentor's connections for invitations. This works particularly well if you are visiting another city for another reason that already covers your expenses. For example, an email enquiry may be productive: *Mary, it was great to chat at the ABC meeting. I will be in San Francisco for a few days the week of 4th April and if possible it would be great to visit your lab. I would also be delighted to give a talk about our work while I'm there if....*

Accepting an invitation carries responsibility: Once you have said yes to an invitation you have several responsibilities. The first is to do the talk. The organizers are relying on you, and the only legitimate reason for canceling a talk is serious illness or some other catastrophe. Backing out of the talk because you are behind on a grant application or because a better offer has come up, is unacceptable. Your second responsibility is to give a decent talk. If you accept an invitation, make sure your mentor knows about it. Most mentors will want to run through the talk to help you put on a good show. When you give a talk, you represent not only yourself but also your mentor.

Be clear you know who pays for what: If you submit an abstract to a scientific meeting and it is accepted for an oral presentation, you will generally have to pay registration and all the costs for attending a meeting. However, if you are invited to speak at a meeting that you would not usually attend, the invitation would usually promise to cover your travel, accommodation, and registration costs. If you visit another institution to give a talk, unless you happen to be in town for another reason, the invitation will almost always cover your expenses.

Sometimes, but more often not, you may get a small honorarium for giving the talk. If you accept the honorarium, remember to declare it with your income taxes.

2. Preparing the content

What are you going to say? The content of your talk will depend on the audience. You would give a different talk about the same topic to medical students and to PhD postdoctoral graduates. When you think about the content of your talk, think about the composition of the audience and how you can keep everybody interested. Many audiences are diverse and can include experts as well as people who know nothing about the topic. You may not be able to keep everybody happy all the time, but you should minimize boredom and maximize interest for everyone.

The big picture is important, the minutiae are stupefying: Remember, you're talking to the whole audience not the one biochemist who understands everything you say before you've said it. Two general rules apply for just about any audience. 1) The big picture is important. Frame the big picture. If everyone in the audience doesn't understand why the topic is critically important, you may as well not give the talk. Too often you will hear scientists launch into their talk about an obscure signaling molecule without telling the audience why it is important. This is a sure way to lose half the audience in the first few sentences of your talk. 2) Remember that although the minutiae, particularly method-ological minutiae, may have taken months to work out and fascinate you and a few cognoscenti, they will stupefy most of the audience. You can only hold the audience if you keep them interested. You do this by weaving a compelling and interesting story, not by dissecting minutiae.

Organizing your content: Most of your talks will combine your work and that of others to tell an interesting story. A story has a beginning, middle, and end. The beginning sets up the background by answering the following questions – why is the topic important, what is known, what is not known, and what is the question you are trying solve. The middle describes the methods and results. The methods section is usually the most boring part of a talk, so focus on the big picture rather than the details. In the results section, a common mistake is to present every result for every experiment. Remember, you're telling a story, not trying to show how much work you've done or how smart you are. The end of the story ties things together nicely and tells the audience what it all means, and what future developments are likely. Some people like to have an outline slide at the beginning of the talk that maps the rest of the talk. That outline slide often reappears before each new subsection of the talk with the next heading highlighted. You can do this if it suits your style, but I find these outline slides tedious. It is more interesting to tell people what you are going to tell them.

Then you start the story and it flows logically from one slide to the next and holds the audience's attention without artificially mapped roadstops.

10 slides or 90 slides do not make a 40 minute talk: Know how long you are expected to speak for. A 1 hour talk usually means 45 minutes of talking, a few minutes for introductions, and 10 minutes at the end for questions. Don't try and squeeze too much information into a talk. If you are asked to speak for 30 minutes, don't take your 60 minute talk and speed up the delivery. If you flash by slides without time to explain them, the audience will not follow your story. Rather, focus on fewer slides that make the important points you want to illustrate. The number of slides you prepare will depend on your speed of delivery and how complex your slides are. For me, 35-40 slides are plenty for a 45 minute talk. Part of rehearsing is to refine the content and speed of your delivery to fit your allotted time. Too few slides are also a problem. The audience will get bored if they are staring at a slide with text they have long since processed. They ask themselves why, if the slide shows everything you want them to remember, are you still talking about it 5 minutes after it has been imprinted in their brains.

Have more data and figure slides and fewer text slides: When a medical student gives a lecture, the talk usually consists of slide after slide of bulleted text that tries to convey the facts needed to pass an exam. This soon becomes boring. You need to be more subtle to entertain your audience. Show them, rather than tell them. If the results of a particular study are important to your argument, show a figure that illustrates the important findings. Rather than a text slide with text that says: The ACCORD study found that 30% of...., show a figure depicting the key findings from ACCORD. The main functions of text slides are to provide a link between figure or table slides and to summarize key points. If more than half your slides are text, you have problem.

3. Preparing the slides

Slides must be clear and error free: Each slide must be crystal clear. This means you have to think about the fonts, text, background, title, figures and tables, and the bells and whistles. Proofread obsessively; spelling mistakes trumpet either your ignorance or sloppiness.

Use big clear fonts: Arial font **36**, 24, 20, 18

There is no point in having a slide that people can't read from the back of the room. I prefer a simple font without curly bits (*sans serif*). In other words, use Arial rather than Times New Roman. If you follow the rule of no more than eight lines of text per slide, and use the biggest font you can, your slides will always be legible. I like 24 font or bigger.

No more than 8 lines of text: Try to have no more than eight lines of text per slide. Obviously there will be exceptions, but it is a good rule of thumb. The text on your slide can be in point form. In other words, what you say will be different from the wording on the slide. There is nothing more boring than listening to a speaker read the exact illegible text from a slide. The words on the slide are there to remind you what you want to say, summarize the main points, and provide an outline for the audience.

The background of the slide should be in the background: The purpose of the slide background is to make your text and other materials more easily visible. In other words, the background provides a contrast to the color of your text. Use the same format on all the slides throughout your talk. Many people use white or yellow text on a blue or another dark colored background, or black text on a white background. There is nothing wrong with using other color combinations, but choose something plain. Creative color contrasts, for example green text on an orange background, come across as amateurish. Generally, avoid red and green because some people are red-green color blind. Backgrounds with multiple colors or designs, or fancy logos are distracting.

The title of the slide should summarize the major point for each slide: It is helpful if the title of each slide summarizes its main point or message. This is helpful to me as I speak because sometimes in the panic of the moment I forget what a particular slide is showing (a sign that I haven't prepared adequately). For example, the title, *Effect of beta-blockers on heart rate*, is vague, whereas *Beta-blockers decrease exercise heart rate* conveys the exact message of the slide. This approach is also helpful to the audience, because if some have fallen asleep, or lost your train of thought, or can't read the figure (a bad mistake on your part), they can glance at the title and get the main message.

Cite your sources: If you use a figure or table from someone else's work to illustrate a point, make sure your slide provides the source. Make sure the citation is legible – someone in the audience might want to refer to the paper. I usually put the first author and the full journal citation but not the title at the bottom of the slide (e.g., Smith AB et al. J Med Bio 2012;12;123-5). Similarly, if the slide shows your own work and it has been published, provide the citation. When you speak about your own work and show data for which you were not primarily responsible, it is good form to give credit to the person who did the experiments. For example, *The figure shows the result of studies in drosophila done by John Smith in our laboratory. As you can see...* Also, if someone shares a slide with you, it is bad form not to acknowledge the person when you are giving your talk.

This is a really busy slide, and I know you can't read it, but... : How many times haven't you heard a speaker show a slide and say something like, *I apologize. This is a really busy slide, and I know you can't read it, but...."* If you ever have to say those words you know you have a lousy slide. Don't apologize, fix the slide. There is no point in showing an illegible figure or table. A common mistake, particularly in basic science talks, is to have four or five figures on the same slide and to expect the audience to work things out for themselves. This is particularly irritating when the speaker only wants to talk about one of the figures. Why not crop the other figures? Similarly, tables can be a nightmare if they are long and illegible. Many of the figures and tables that you download as slides from prominent journals are illegible when you project them.

Omit the bells and whistles: The software programs for making slides allow speakers to do too many creative things. Restrain yourself and stick to simple slides with no or minimal animation, a plain background, no catchy drawings, icons or logos from the library of illustrations, and no exclamation points! If you must show a video from a slide, make sure the video works on the system in the room where you are giving the talk.

Cute slides: Some speakers can mix a few joke slides seamlessly into their talks and come across as polished and entertaining. The danger is that humor can fall flat and you come across like a stand-up comic with a silent audience. There is no rule that you have to give a funny scientific talk, although some humor can keep the audience engaged. Until you are a veteran speaker and can read your audience well, avoid slides unrelated to the content of your talk. This includes slides of your children, spouse, pets, holiday, or favorite sport.

Some examples of problem slides:

Slides: The Bad, Bad Slide

Background: Free fatty acids (FFAs) affect insulin signaling and are implicated in the pathogenesis of insulin resistance and atherosclerosis. Inflammatory cytokines such as interleukin-6 (IL-6) increase lipolysis and thus levels of FFAs.

We hypothesized that increased IL-6 concentrations are associated with increased FFAs resulting in insulin resistance and atherosclerosis in rheumatoid arthritis (RA) and designed the study that I will describe fully next.

Problems
Fuzzy font title, text too small, too much text, written for reading not speaking.

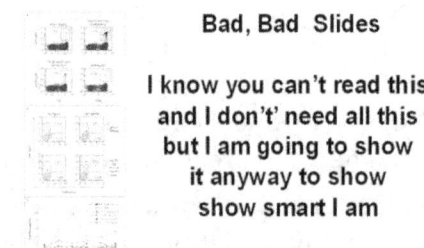

Bad, Bad Slides

I know you can't read this and I don't' need all this but I am going to show it anyway to show show smart I am

Problems
Downloaded from a journal where it makes a beautiful figure this is a poor slide because it is illegible and takes too long to explain.

Bad, Bad Slides :

Problems
A table downloaded from a journal can make a poor slide because it is illegible and takes too long to explain.

4. Preparing the delivery

Preparing the words: Preparing a talk is not just about having interesting information and making clear slides, it is also about preparing your delivery. Your preparation should be meticulous. Part of preparing is to decide what you are going to say. I like to write the exact text of what I plan to say for each slide. This script helps me focus on the message of each slide and choose words that carry my message most effectively. It also stops me saying stupid things and rambling, which I do when I speak on the fly. I don't try and memorize the exact words, nor do I try to read or refer to my script when I'm giving the actual talk. I find that after many rehearsals most of the wording sticks in my head. Your script should be in "spoken English" rather than "written English." In other words, cutting and pasting the text from a paper that you've written and memorizing or reading it is not a good idea, because that's not the way we talk. We speak more directly, casually, and in shorter sentences than we write.

Transition between slides – "now to change gears completely" wrecks the engine: The slide is the unit of information, and when you put all the units in order they should link to tell your story. If you've done a good job, the story flows seamlessly as the slides roll. This takes preparation, because there is always a transition between the current slide and the next. This transition is the least intuitive part of preparing a talk. You know what you want to say for each slide, but what takes more work is finding the words that link the slides so that the story flows. You will find that when you are rehearsing aloud you realize the story is not flowing and that perhaps you need to move a slide, add a slide, delete a slide, or change what you say to improve the flow. *Now to change gears completely* is not a transition; it is a lazy way of apologizing for not linking the story.

Rehearse, rehearse, rehearse: I will never forget walking past an empty lecture hall where someone was giving a talk. It was one of the most prominent scientists at our institution, a seasoned speaker, who was rehearsing a talk aloud in an empty hall. I had always thought that experienced speakers could shuffle their slide deck a few minutes ahead of time and then give a great talk on the fly.

What I've learned is that it takes a lot of work and rehearsal for most people to give a good talk.

Rehearse aloud: When you start to practice, do so at your desk in front of your computer. Once you're close to a final product, rehearse standing, talking aloud, with your slides in the full screen presentation format, and using a pointer. This allows you to practice when, and more important, when not to use the pointer. The pointer should stay in its holster unless needed. The audience does not need the pointer to read simple text slides. The pointer is for directing the audience to a specific number, or a feature on a figure that you are describing. In addition to pointer practice, another benefit of practicing aloud is that you can develop the nuances of timing your delivery. You sense when to speed up because the talk is getting boring and when to slow down because the concept is difficult. You also learn to associate each slide with its keys points and potential delivery problems.

Rehearse with a tame audience: Once you are happy with the talk and your delivery, find a few people to be a tame audience and listen to you, ideally in the same room where you will give the real talk. Give your talk uninterrupted, just as you plan to deliver it. Then ask your critics to comment on the slides and their legibility from the back of the room, the content, and your delivery. Also, ask them to predict questions that the audience might ask.

5. The delivery

Dress professionally: Look professional; don't overdress or underdress.

Bring the right technology (and your slides): When you accept an invitation to give a talk make sure you know what technology you will need. Should you bring your own computer? If so, is it compatible? Should you bring a thumb drive? Even if you have emailed your slides to the organizer ahead of time, take a spare copy on a thumb drive (and also email a copy of your presentation to yourself) as backup. On several occasions I have emailed my slides to the organizer of an event with the arrangement they would be preloaded and ready to roll, only to enter the room and be greeted with, "OK, can I have your slides?"

Bring your own pointer: How many times have you seen a speaker struggle with a laser pointer that did not work, was difficult to manage, or was so feeble no one could see it? Bring your own pointer. Buy one with a bright signal.

Scout the podium: Arrive in good time so that you can load your talk and run through your slides very quickly. It is embarrassing when a slide that was perfect on your computer, now projects with all the symbols for the Greek letter alpha replaced by eyeglass icons. Also, use these few minutes to walk up to the podium and learn where the stairs are. At the podium, test the controls. Learn how to turn the microphone on, load your talk after the previous speaker has finished, advance the slides, and to work the pointer. It is embarrassing when the first sentences of a talk are, "Now, how do I dim the lights….can I have the first slide please….oh, I do the slides…is this the button for the first slide…. is there a pointer?"

Use the microphone: Turn off your cell phone and pager, and if there is a clip-on microphone make sure that it does not rub on your clothing or jewelry. Cell phones often interfere with microphones – I put my cell phone on the podium, a long way from the microphone. Don't try to talk without the microphone. Some speakers seem to believe that it is a sign of weakness or incompetence to use a microphone in a medium-sized room. They make a show of not needing the microphone, and unfortunately the audience suffers. The microphone is usually there for a reason.

Meet the chair and stay close: If you are talking at a session where there is a chairperson, arrive early and introduce yourself so that the chair knows you have arrived and learns how to pronounce your name. Once your talk is loaded, and you are familiar with the podium controls, choose a seat close to the stage so that you don't have to fight your way across a row of seats on your way to the podium. Unless you never burp, don't drink sodas before the talk.

Everyone is nervous: As you sit in your chair listening to the preceding speakers, you will be nervous. Remind yourself that everyone is nervous no matter how many talks they have given. If nerves are a problem, you will have to find a way to deal with them. Giving a lot of talks is a good way. So too is rehearsing a lot. It helps me to write out the first two sentences of my talk on a piece of paper to jog my memory out of its frozen state at the podium. Another helpful technique to quell the nerves is to remind yourself that most people give a lousy talk and you know yours will not be bad because you have rehearsed it to perfection. Also, recognizing that giving a talk is just part of what we do – this is just another part of the job – can help. I have not found that the recommended techniques of imagining the audience to be naked or focusing your gaze on a familiar face in the audience help me, but you might. Any nervous tremor you have will be magnified on the screen by the pointer. To minimize advertising your nervousness, you can avoid using the pointer during the first part of the talk when you are most nervous, or you can hold the pointer with two hands to keep it steady.

Deliver: The first few minutes of a talk are the most important. Your approval ratings start high, and the audience will listen for short time in a nonjudgmental way; this is your best chance to engage them. When you arrive at the podium, first organize yourself. Stand up straight, get your title slide up, clip the microphone on, and get the pointer working. Then, when you are ready, look at the audience confidently, breathe, smile, <u>pause</u>, and then ready, steady, go. That little pause is a magic moment. The orchestra is poised, the audience is silent, and you, the conductor, are about to start a symphony. The opening few sentences of your talk should hook the audience. Design your talk so that the first few sentences grab the audience's attention without being corny or dramatic.

Delivery is easy: The delivery of your talk is the easiest part. You've prepared, refined your content, slides, and script, and rehearsed many times. Now two things are important: 1) to be audible, and 2) not to irritate the audience.

Make eye contact with members of the audience at the back of the room. If someone there is holding a hand to his ear – take note and action. If you are uncertain whether people can hear you, then ask. Being audible is easy, not being irritating is difficult; we all have mannerisms, often without knowing about them. It can be illuminating, not to say deflating, to videotape yourself giving a talk. Here are some irritating habits to avoid.

1. Speaking to the screen and not the audience.
2. Reading from a script or from the slides.
3. Not varying the pace of your delivery or tone of voice.
4. Using slang or jargon. Nothing is "cool" or "sexy" about those words.
5. Verbal tics such as um, umm, and you know, you know.
6. Physical tics such as rocking, slumping, swaying, fiddling, tapping, and picking.
7. Waving the pointer across the screen like a demented conductor.
8. Pointing at every word on the screen.
9. Shining the pointer at the audience.
10. Fiddling with the microphone to produce a viscerally unpleasant cacophony.
11. Going backwards to previous slides to make a point. If your talk demands that you go back to a slide, rather insert a copy of that slide into your lineup.
12. Running over time.

Delivery is not always easy: No matter how well prepared you are, or how extensively you test the technology, things can still go wrong. We have all been at talks where the speaker knocks over a glass of water, the projector's bulb blows, the computer crashes, the screen turns black, the microphone has feedback like an electric guitar, the slides project unbidden in random order, and so on. If you give enough talks, some of these things will happen to you. For the audience, the talk has been replaced by the much more entertaining spectacle of you panicking. This is a time for "grace under pressure" (Ernest Hemingway's definition of "guts"). If you don't panic (easier said than done) and are prepared to laugh at the situation and yourself, the audience will stop sniggering at your discomfort and wait comfortably for someone to fix the technology. If it can't be fixed within a reasonable time, you might have to retire to fight another day unless you are confident you can give a reasonable talk without the slides.

A patient, or a person you criticize, may be in the audience: You can never tell who will be in the audience. Therefore, it is important to be sensitive and diplomatic. If you are talking about a medical condition, remember that there may be patients with that condition in the audience. "This is a really terrible disease with a horrible prognosis," is insensitive. Jokes or derogatory comments about a disease that are meant to be funny are crass ("I hide under my desk when I see patients with xy, they are high maintenance, always whining…"). Also, remember that the authors of the work you discuss may be in the audience. "I don't really believe these data…" or, "This was a really lousy experiment…" or, "We could not reproduce these data no matter how hard we tried….." are fighting words.

"No sinner is ever saved after the first 20 minutes of a sermon" (Mark Twain): People almost never complain that a talk was too short. If you finish a few minutes early, most of the audience will be delighted. It will give them time to get to their appointments, catch up on email, or reflect on what a wonderful talk you gave. Make sure you keep track of time and allow for questions and discussion. If you ever find yourself in the position of having used your whole hour and saying, "I know we are over time. Would you like me to go on, I've almost finished?" you need a reality check. No one ever wants speakers to continue after their allocated hour – never, ever.

Plan an exit strategy if you are running out of time: Sometimes, even with the best planning, your timing can be off. The talk can start late, the introduction can be long, and members of the audience might interrupt during the talk to ask questions. If you find yourself running out of time, don't feel you have to apologize and go as fast as you can. Rather, have a planned exit strategy and summarize the last four or five slides that you are going to skip in a sentence or two. Say something like, "I want to leave some time for questions. These few slides that I am going to skip over show…" and then move onto your conclusion slide and finish gracefully. If you are giving a talk and have mistimed things and find yourself 5-10 minutes from the end with several slides to go, activate your exit strategy and get to the conclusion slide rapidly. If you don't, the audience will become increasingly restive as the end of your allocated time approaches, and you will become increasingly harried if you try and squeeze everything into the last few minutes.

"To conclude this part of talk…:" The only slide that should have the word "conclusion" in the heading is your second-last slide. It is painful to be bored out of one's wits, see a slide with the word "conclusion" and rejoice inwardly, only to have the speaker say, "To conclude this part of the talk…" and then drone on.

Conclusion: The conclusion slide is usually your second last slide, and you use it to repeat the main messages. Speakers often make the mistake of losing steam and reading the text of the conclusion slide quickly like a religious incantation, mumbling in a sing-song voice. In reality, it is one of the most important slides in your talk. When the audience sees the heading "Conclusion," they perk up, and some (often the chair) decide what questions they can ask. Look at the audience and elevate your energy and enthusiasm during the conclusion slide.

Acknowledgements: The last slide is usually the acknowledgements slide. It should include the names (pictures can be nice) of the people who contributed to the work you presented. It should also list the grant funding that supported the work. Sometimes, speakers sound as though they are giving an Academy Award acceptance speech, thanking everyone listed on the slide individually in great detail. I prefer to say a couple of sentences for this slide and not to go into details about who did what. During your talk, when you show a data slide, you can mention the contributions of a particular person. After you have acknowledged your collaborators, thank the audience, and offer to take questions.

Question time is risky: Questions are risky and you are most vulnerable because you are not in control of the agenda and anyone could ask a question that exposes your ignorance or a flaw in your study. Remember, most people are not trying to put you down. Also, you can decrease the risk with good preparation.

Prepare for the obvious: For some talks (e.g., presenting an abstract at a meeting), there will always be questions if you finish a few minutes early, as you should. The chairperson has to keep proceedings on a strict schedule to allow members of the audience to move between talks in different rooms. If only to fill time, the chair will ask some obvious, softball question. For example, "What are the clinical implications of your findings?"; "Can you expand a little on your comment that……?" (and refer to something on one of your last few slides); "Is there an animal/human/cell/knockout model that could be informative?" Prepare responses for the obvious icebreaker questions. Your presentation will generate some predictable questions – ask your practice audience to pepper you with questions. Prepare scripted answers to these. You can keep extra slides in reserve that illustrate some of these points, but generally, unless the point is complex, it is more trouble than it is worth to navigate to the extra slide.

What if no one asks a question? Some people suggest that if no one asks a question you should ask the first question yourself. I find it odd when a speaker does this. If no one asks a question I usually thank the audience and close the session. A lack of questions may reflect an audience that is overwhelmed, bored, fully informed, replete, intimidated, shy, uninterested, disconnected, happy, hungry, or focused on the next engagement. Make sure you ask some members of an audience that did not ask you any questions for feedback.

"That is a very good question:" Don't interrupt when someone is asking a question. When the person is finished, many speakers say, "That is a really good question." If they say it in response to every question it seems insincere; if they only say it for some questions, it implies that the other questions were not so good. Rather than praise the question, say, "Thank you, the question is..." and then repeat or rephrase the question, because the rest of the audience may not have heard it. Rephrasing the question also gives you time to organize your thoughts. Then answer the question with a polite and relatively short response. You should answer most questions in a couple of sentences. Stop yourself from rambling into related areas in an attempt to fill time and forestall additional questions or because your adrenalin is still flowing.

"Your study was underpowered:" If a comment or question criticizes an element of your study, it is important not to collapse, roll over, and join the questioner in disemboweling yourself by saying something like this: "Yes, you are absolutely right, our study was very small and underpowered, and to make matters worse the data are noisy because 2 people did not adhere to therapy." Don't fall on your sword. Even if the comment is correct, emphasize the positive. For example, "The study was indeed relatively small, but it is worth noting that despite the small sample size, perhaps because we controlled for confounding factors meticulously, responses in the two groups were significantly different." If there are obvious weaknesses in your study, it is wise to mention them in your talk and shore up your defenses preemptively.

Gobsmacked: What if someone asks you a question that you have no idea how to answer? There are several options – the least satisfactory is to get a deer-in-the-headlights look, scan the room for your mentor like a drowning person, and play for time by asking the person to repeat the question. What may happen then is that the person restates the question, now in terms so clear that a 3rd grader can understand it, and you are in an even worse position. Another option is to answer that you don't know and leave it at that. This is reasonable if the question is esoteric, but is embarrassing if you should know the answer. If the elusive answer is in your data and you can look it up, say that you don't remember the exact numbers or details but can find the answer after the talk. Another option for dealing with difficult questions is to say you don't have a direct answer, but... and then launch into an answer that is somewhat related to the area of the question. Politicians do this all the time and call it "staying on message." Most people who ask questions will realize that you are on the defense and will retire gracefully and let you salvage your dignity. Similarly, if someone asks a question that you think is stupid because you already explained it extensively in your talk, answer the question in a way that maintains the dignity of the questioner: "Thank you. The question is whether... It is worth emphasizing that one of our main findings was that... and the implications of this are..."

Never lose your cool: Be calm, pleasant, and confident. Don't argue with someone in the audience, no matter how aggressive or wrong the person is. Defuse the situation by pleasantly acknowledging the questioner's opinion, diplomatically stating your position, and acknowledging different opinions. For example, "Thank you. The possibility that.... (summarize what the questioner said) is an interesting point of view. I see it somewhat differently... (say what you think), but there are obviously different opinions."

6. The postmortem

Keep tweaking your talk: It is a good idea to keep modifying your talk and slides. The best time to do this is immediately after you have given the talk. Your memory of which slides worked and which did not, where the talk dragged, and where the audience became restive is fresh. You can (and should) give the same talk many times. So it is a good idea to keep tweaking it – no matter how many times you have given it. Also, if you know someone in the audience, ask for feedback. (Remember to ask for ways to improve the talk next time, not for criticism of today's talk.) People generally won't offer you feedback spontaneously because it could be viewed as criticism, but if you ask directly, you will get constructive suggestions.

Update your CV: Remember to update your CV after you have given a talk, particularly one outside your institution.

Summary

Giving talks – don't do this:	Giving talks – do this:
Turn invitations down	Invite invitations to talk
Start ineptly	Do them
Mumble	Prepare obsessively
Read endless slides	Rehearse out loud
Get lost	Rehearse with a tame audience
Go back to a previous slide	Keep it simple and short
Paint with the pointer	Check your slides in slideshow format
Bore or irritate the audience	Check the podium and technology
Show the audience your back	Prepare for questions
Run over time	Record talks on your CV
Have illegible slides	Keep tweaking your talk

Resources

1. Scientifically Speaking: Tips for preparing and delivering scientific talks and using visual aids. The Oceanographic Society, 2005. https://tos.org/pdfs/sci_speaking.pdf

2. The Northwestern University Collaborative Learning and Integrated Mentoring in the Biosciences (CLIMB) website has several resources for speakers. http://www.northwestern.edu/climb/resources/oral-communication-skills/creating-a-presentation.html

Chapter 25

Avoid an email mess

How people get into trouble with email

Communication by email is wonderful, but can get you into trouble. There is a short, entertaining book: *SEND: Why People Email So Badly and How to Do It Better* by David Shipley and Will Schwalbe (1) that everyone who uses email should read. It describes email etiquette and common problems; many of the points in this chapter come from the book. Problems with email often occur for the following reasons.

1. Inappropriate information.
2. Inappropriate tone.
3. Inappropriate recipients.
4. Replying or not replying.
5. Using email to solve a serious problem.
6. Not keeping important emails.
7. Careless errors and lack of consideration.

1. Inappropriate information

Confidentiality: You cannot expect an email to be confidential – your employer and the person receiving the email have no obligation to respect your privacy. Most employers reserve the right to monitor all activities on their computers and networks, including private communications sent to personal email addresses. For example, the Food and Drug Administration monitored the communications of several employees, including their personal emails and documents on personal thumb drives (2). Also, the recipient of your email can send it to anyone, including the very person you did not want to see the email. Don't write an email you wouldn't want published in the *New York Times* (mentor Alastair Wood).

Potentially damaging statements: Email leaves a permanent record that you cannot control. There are many examples of subpoenaed emails that became part of legal action. You should assume that anything you write in an email could end up in court. An email is not the place for speculation that could be quoted out of context. For example, John has just sent you preliminary data from an animal cancer experiment. Here is an email you dash off and cc the whole laboratory: *John, Thanks for the data on AB123. This is a fantastic cure rate but*

I have grave concerns about the toxicity data. There is a huge market for the drug but it may kill as many people as it cures. We need to do something with these data. Mike

The email has many problems. It reflects your unprocessed thoughts and speculates wildly about future scenarios. You can imagine how 10 years later your email could be interpreted as strong evidence that this drug should never have been given to humans. Also worrying in the email is your mention of the market (implying that marketing strengths may trump safety weaknesses), and your suggestion that "we need to do something with the data" (bury it? falsify it?). It was also unnecessary to copy the email to the whole laboratory. A better response would be short, bland, polite, and businesslike: *John, Thanks for the data on AB123. We need to sit down and plan the next studies. Mike*

Too much information: An email should be short and focus on one topic or question. Busy people get hundreds of emails a day and often stop reading after the first question. The second question you ask may be invisible.

Everyone can see everything: People often add their responses to the original email and the string of previous responses. This is convenient because you can review all the communications in one email and eventually you need save only the final email. Different people join the string at different stages and problems occur when there is sensitive information (e.g., details about salaries) buried in previous emails that is not meant for some of the people who joined the string later.

Subject and body mismatch: Sometimes an email string keeps a subject line that is no longer related to the body of the email. For example, I invite John to lunch with the subject line *Lunch on Thursday* and he responds but adds a question about the results of a study. I then request the results of the study from someone else by forwarding John's email that still has the subject line *Lunch on Thursday*. An email with a mismatch between the subject line and its body is confusing, easy to misunderstand, and difficult to find when you are searching for it.

2. Inappropriate tone or content

Open to interpretation: How do you interpret this email: *This is an unbelievable paper.*? It could mean that the paper is unbelievably good, or unbelievably bad, or that the results are wrong or fabricated. In conversation, your tone would clarify your meaning; in an email, your words stand alone. Avoid sending emails that could be misinterpreted. The easiest way to do that is to keep your tone cordial, bland, and businesslike.

Emoticons!!! If you need to add smiley faces or sad faces to your emails to make sure they are not misunderstood, you are either communicating information that should not be communicated by email, or you are communicating about a potentially touchy topic with people who do not know you well enough to recognize what you intend to say. Both are potentially dangerous situations. Keep emails bland. If you feel the need to reach for an emoticon, regard it as a warning flag. Similarly, other than for congratulations, a need for exclamation marks suggests too much emotion for email!!! ☺☺

Anger: Venting by email may feel good, but if you are angry do not write an email. You will say things that are inflammatory, counterproductive, and permanent. You should not try to resolve a problem that makes you angry by email. Rather, talk to the person when you have cooled down and had time to work out a strategy. Avoid all caps, it suggests ANGER.

Sarcasm: Sarcasm communicates criticism or humor; neither is appropriate for email.

Humor: Business email is for business; never send or forward jokes or cartoons. What one person finds funny, another may find racist, sexist, demeaning, or rude. Don't use humor in your own emails, unless you know the recipient extremely well, and even then, avoid humor related to sex, religion, politics, ethnicity, gender, population group, and just about any other topic, other than poking fun at yourself.

Hey buddy, Hi Mike – inappropriate salutation: I receive many enquiries from strangers enquiring about a postdoctoral position in my group that start off, *Hi Mike*. If you don't know a person well, the safest email salutation is formal, e.g., *Dear Dr. X*. If Dr. X then signs an email with a first name, it is reasonable for you to respond using the first name. If the response is signed with first and last names, continue with *Dear Dr. X*. The term "Dear" is falling out of fashion in emails. People debate the best alternative. A bland "Good morning" or "Good afternoon" followed by the person's name is acceptable, but is less formal than "Dear." Only use "Hi" for people you know.

Inappropriate content: Content that is not about business is not suitable for a business email account. This includes humor, politics, gossip, your social life, etc.

Inappropriate email address: Most academic centers allocate you a standard email address based on a permutation of your name. If you create a private email account, make sure your address is bland, based on your name, and does not contain words that that convey emotion (love, hate, happy), attempted humor (party animal, slacker), or anything else (smartestdoc, researchbeast, mensa-member).

Inappropriate fonts and additions: Us a bland, readable, 11 or 12-point black font such as Arial, Calibri, or Times New Roman. Don't embellish your email signature with aphorisms, interesting quotations, pithy religious or political thoughts, uplifting phrases, or anything other than your name, title, and contact information.

3) Inappropriate recipients

to: We all receive too many emails. Each recipient of your email should have a reason to receive it.

cc: As the supervisor of a project, I do not like to receive copies of every piece of correspondence related to the project. But I do want to hear about important things; it is up to mentees to use judgment. Be careful. If you never cc your boss on an email string and then you suddenly do, it sends the message that you are unhappy with the performance of the recipient and are now copying your boss as a threat or an unspoken message of dissatisfaction.

bcc: I prefer not to blind copy emails, and if need be, rather forward a copy of the email directly with a note explaining why I forwarded it. Be very careful; forwarding an email without asking, copying, or telling the sender is sneaky.

4) Replying or not replying

Reply: If I ask something, you should answer; if I send something that you asked for, you should say thank you; however, you are not obliged to answer every email. Sometimes email strings with repeated variations on the theme of "thank you" or "I agree" become ludicrous.

Reply all: Before you automatically hit "reply all," decide who needs to see your response and be doubly careful what you say. For example, many journal editors will send the rejection letter to all co-authors. If you hit "reply all" to send a note of frustration to all your co-authors (*This idiotic journal has published so much rubbish lately it is not surprising they cannot recognize good work when they see it!!)* your email will also go to the editor.

Time to reply: Be consistent in the time you take to reply to an email. If you are one of those people who responds within minutes, people will expect a quick reply, and if you do not reply for a day or two, it sends the message that you have demoted the person or the problem.

Not replying: There are some people who do not reply to emails, even ones asking a direct question. Sometimes this is accidental – an email is deleted or placed in the wrong folder, but often it is deliberate. If you ignore people, it sends the message that they are not important to you. It is interesting that the people who ignore your emails are often the very ones who expect an instant reply when they send an email and want something.

5) Using email to solve a serious problem

I hate what you are doing: If you have a problem with a colleague, trying to deal with it by email will often make it worse. Compared to conversation, email is a poor tool for nuanced communication. In a conversation you can modify the content and tone of what you say based on cues from the other person. I find it incredible when a postdoc who works 3 benches from another prints me a series of increasingly heated email exchanges to show what a problem the other person is. Most problems arise from conflicting needs or expectations and are opportunities to learn to negotiate. Walk across the hall and talk to someone.

6) Not keeping important emails

What did we decide? Increasingly, emails are records of events. Many institutions do not allow you to have an infinitely large inbox. Make folders to organize the emails you wish to keep. You should keep important emails, for example those that document a decision or agreement. Sometimes, after a conversation I send an informal email of thanks that summarizes the discussion so that I have a written and dated record for my file. For example, *John, Great talking to you today. I am so appreciative that your company can provide the 50 BP monitors we need for our study free of charge. This will help us a lot. Much appreciated. Mike.* Sometimes, I send an email note to myself to remind me (and have a permanent record) of what happened in a conversation, particularly a difficult conversation.

7) Careless errors and lack of consideration

Some people believe that it is a waste of time to correct spelling errors in emails and that sending an email with errors is, in fact, evidence of your excellent time utilization. I disagree. An email full of errors makes you look sloppy and ignorant. Read your emails carefully for errors – they can be embarrassing. An administrator checking my credentials once sent me an email asking if he could use Dr. X as a reference. I meant to respond, *Yes, I previously used him,* but what I typed (and sent) was, *Yes, I previously sued him.* Spelling autocorrect options can cause unintentional embarrassing changes. Here are some that nearly embarrassed me: warfarin – warfare, omics – comics, PGRN – PORN, Pubmed – Plumbed, terfenadine – turpentine, DSMB – DUMB.

DON'T SHOUT: If you feel the need to use all caps in an email to make a point, it suggests that email is NOT THE APPROPRIATE WAY to communicate.

Don't respond to listserv emails or responses: When you reply to a message sent to a group of people on a listserv, your reply (even if you hit "reply" and not "reply all") might go to everyone on that listserv, depending on the way the message and list were set up. Rather, send a separate email with your response to the person who sent the original email. If you are the recipient of an email from someone who responded to a list serve, do not reply. Your reply, and all the other replies, will be sent to everyone on the list creating what is termed an email storm (3) that can overwhelm the system.

Summary

1. Keep emails short, cordial, bland, and about business.

2. Avoid criticism, jokes, and emotion.

3. Don't try to solve serious problems by email.

4. Assume your email will be forwarded to anyone and everyone.

5. There is no need to respond to some emails.

6. There is no need to always copy a crowd.

7. Imagine any email you send published in the *New York Times.*

Resources

1. SEND: Why People Email So Badly and How to Do It Better, by David Shipley and Will Schwalbe, Vintage 2010.

2. Article in the *New York Times* July 14, 2012 describing how the Food and Drug Administration monitored the communications of employees. http://www.nytimes.com/2012/07/15/us/fda-surveillance-of-scientists-spread-to-outside-critics.html?_r=0

3. Email storms. http://en.wikipedia.org/wiki/Email_storm

Chapter 26
Leadership, collaboration, and good citizenship

Leadership

Leadership at an academic institution: At an academic institution everyone is a leader to some extent. For example, even as a trainee you might lead a project and direct students. Some individuals, however, rise to lead divisions, departments, centers, teaching or service groups, and institutions. At the beginning of your academic career it may seem premature to be thinking about leadership, but it is important to consider your long-term goals. If a senior leadership position is one of your goals, it will require specific skills, training, and work.

Leadership traits: Many think that the best scientists are the people that rise to academic leadership positions. This is often not the case. The very characteristics that make good a scientist – self-doubt, criticism, skepticism, contrarian thinking, focus, creativity, and perfectionism – can be a hindrance to a leader. Leadership and science require different sets of skills; both can be learnt.

Many books on leadership discuss various attributes of a leader; for example – focus, vision, integrity, ruthlessness, willingness to take risk, reliability, optimism, realism, energetic, reflective, individualistic, team builder, shrewd, generous, hands-on, delegates, humble, confident, listens to others, marches to own drum, passionate, rational, consistent, thinks out-of-the-box, flexible, decisive, logical and intuitive. Superficially, these leadership traits all seem reasonable, even though many are direct opposites. However, they don't describe three characteristics that are the crux of leadership: 1) behavior; 2) following; and 3) results.

*1) **Leaders behave like leaders:*** Aspiring leaders, consciously or subconsciously want to be leaders and behave in the following ways:

- They associate with leaders and potential leaders, not necessarily in a sycophantic way, because it helps create a path to leadership. Aspiring leaders often seek each other out, sit together, show mutual respect, and support each other.
- They realize that leaders bring positive energy and do not vent, complain, or show anger, negativity, or frustration. They are careful

what they say. Aspiring leaders seldom show much of a sense of humor in public – jokes or funny asides usually require spontaneity and have the potential to offend, be misinterpreted, or come across as negative. If you have a sarcastic, critical, or loose tongue, the first step towards leadership is to develop new filters.

- They understand that leaders are visible, do not rock the institutional boat, and do not make unnecessary enemies. Therefore, they avoid confrontation and find positive ways to solve problems and suggest direction.
- They recognize that leaders move ideas (not necessarily their own) forward to benefit the institution. Therefore, they align themselves with people and initiatives that are important to the institution.
- They understand that the total package is important. Their dress, speech, and behavior inside and outside work all reflect the leaders they want to be.

*2) **Leaders are good followers:*** Leadership is hierarchical, and even the most senior leader is answerable to a higher-ranking leader or group. This means that every leader has to be a good follower. Once an institution has made decisions, leaders accept and implement them, even those they disagree with, efficiently and positively, without criticism. If you do not share the vision of your leader, you are part of the problem. Usually you have little to gain and a lot to lose by fighting with your boss.

*3) **Leaders get results:*** Leaders have the difficult task of acting in the best interests of a group while any particular action they take will not always be in the best interests of each individual member. Leaders are judged by their results, and perhaps surprisingly for a community focused on science, the commonest metric is a unit's finances (e.g., grant or clinical income). Leaders get results in different ways: by inspiring, empowering, hiring, firing, coaching, doing nothing, being lucky, persuading, encouraging, supporting, educating, nagging, manipulating, trading, rewarding, prodding, bribing, and threatening. Generally, a leader's results are more important than the process by which they are obtained, unless the process harms the institution. Therefore, leaders are not necessarily popular or nice people; however, the best leaders lead and get results in ways that engender support, respect, and commitment to a common vision.

Becoming a leader: In the early stages of your development it is much more important to focus on your academic career than seek leadership opportunities. Nevertheless, even if you think you will never want to be a leader, it is a good idea to learn to behave like one. Not only will leadership behavior keep that career option open for you, but your research career will also benefit. Read books on leadership and consider taking some classes (many business schools offer them).

Aspiring leaders often start the road to leadership by carving out a small project and making a success of it; for example, starting a new program that fills an institutional need or taking over an existing program. These endeavors require time, effort, and political skills; make sure the program is close to your heart, that you are committed to its success, and that your science does not suffer.

Talking to leaders: Leaders don't whine. Whining or venting is complaining about problems without proposing a feasible solution. We all feel better after a good whine, and a friend will listen to you complain and then commiserate and pat you on the back. But do not mistake a friendly leader for a friend. If you vent to a leader, you can come across as negative, unappreciative of the support given to you, not worth investing in, and critical of current leadership. When you subsequently approach the leader for support (e.g., promotion, a startup package) your negotiation is affected by your previous baring of your soul that you thought was just a heart-to-heart chat. You can vent to trustworthy mentors (even if they are leaders); their job is to teach you to either find a solution or to stop complaining about something that cannot be fixed. You cannot vent to subordinates, it is bad for morale and for your reputation. Venting feels good but is dangerous because it is negative, stuck in the past, and self-sustaining. A mentoring approach that I learnt from my daughter Zoe can break the cycle of venting. She once said to me, "Are you venting or do you want advice. If you are venting you've got 2 minutes, then you get my advice." As a mentor, I focus my advice on solving the problem or moving on if it is not soluble.

The right time for a leadership position: It is prudent to wait until your career is established and you have been promoted to associate professor before taking on a leadership role. Although it is flattering, be wary of accepting a leadership position too early. Leadership involves service to others and requires time and energy. Each position has a limited lifespan. Institutions sometimes offer leadership positions to attract young faculty at the cutting edge of research. For example, Dr. A is a young assistant professor with five *Nature* papers and three RO1's and is attracted to an institution by the offer of leadership of a small division. Then, as 15 years go by, what was an exciting area of research has become run-of-the-mill, and Dr. A has not published in *Nature* again and is struggling to keep one RO1. The institution wants to attract new blood with the offer of leadership of the division. Dr. A is asked to step down to "focus on the lab," or to move to a position with more administrative duties. One of the reasons Dr. A has not lived up to potential is that leadership makes substantial demands on time and energy. Think ahead, if you are offered the directorship of a division at the age of 35, are you planning to hold the position for 30 years until you retire? If not, what will your next job be?

Leadership – recognizing the silent coup: Academic politics is generally easy to understand and is driven by recognizable personality types and the confluence of institutional and self-interest. Not so obvious is a political process you should know about – change of leadership by silent coup. From the outside the process looks like evolutionary change and it avoids public discord. It goes like this. The chief decides to bring in a more favored leader (person B) without firing or demoting the current leader (person A). The chief asks B to "assist" A with specific components of the program. The chief and B then progressively sideline A by changing the focus of the program in B's direction, meeting and making decisions without including A, and slowly moving responsibilities to B. After a while, it is clear that B is the *de facto* leader. Person A has relatively few options: 1) to step down and make the change official, 2) to continue in an untenable position until the chief makes the change official, 3) to confront the chief and B and appear paranoid, 4) to speak to the chief about a carving out something new. Avoid situations in which you are either person A or person B.

Collaboration

Be a good collaborator – show up and be considerate: You will need to collaborate to do good science and have a successful career. Small things make a big impression. For example, when I have new collaborators on a grant it is a bad sign if I have trouble getting them to send a biosketch with an appropriate personal statement, or they do not make useful comments about the grant. A good collaborator has two key characteristics: showing up and being considerate. Showing up means you are reliable, you attend meetings or teleconferences (or apologize if you cannot attend), you engage in the project fully, and you respond promptly to emails related to the collaboration. Being considerate means that you do your fair share of the work, you do it well and with enthusiasm, and you treat your collaborators as you would like to be treated. No one wants a collaborator who works slowly and reluctantly, does not respond to communications, misses deadlines, does not do a fair share of the work, and tries to take credit unfairly. When you are the new person joining an established group you should be sensitive to the existing group dynamics and modulate your style accordingly.

Be a good collaborator – respect primate behavior: Food, territory, and hierarchical rank are strong driving forces for primate behavior. The same forces apply in academic medicine. People are rewarded with money (food), space (territory), and rank (titles, achievements). Respect these when you deal with other academics. Scouting out someone's lab (that looks underutilized) with a tape measure will not make you popular. Using someone's space or equipment without permission is asking for trouble. It is important to acknowledge the contributions of collaborators in talks and to credit them with appropriate authorship on papers.

Choose collaborators well – good scientists and good collaborators who are in your zone: Choose to collaborate with people who are not only good scientists but also good collaborators. If you are thinking of collaborating with someone, look them up in PubMed, because a non-productive past career is likely to lead to a non-productive collaboration. Choose collaborations that are likely to succeed, but keep in mind that the outcome of collaboration is never predictable and some projects die. Collaborative work should fall inside your broad zone of focus or diversification. Random collaborations show lack of focus. You can collaborate up, down, and sideways. Each direction has different challenges.

Choose good collaborators – collaborating up: Collaborating with investigators senior to you can pose particular challenges. You might find it hard to set boundaries in terms of the work they ask you to do and to assert yourself when credit is allocated. It is important to communicate early.

Choose good collaborators – collaborating down: You are likely to mentor students, residents, and fellows; they become your collaborators. Be careful if the focus is "to get an abstract" rather than to learn how to be a scientist. Make sure you do not overextend your resources by taking on too many beginner researchers for one-off projects; do not invest in people who are merely going through the motions to get a better clinical position.

Choose good collaborators – collaborating sideways: Collaborating with a peer can be tricky because you are both on the same rung of the career ladder. You both need your own grants and first or last author papers. Again, good early communication about these questions is important.

Problems with collaborators: Most problems with collaborators arise because people have differences in flexibility or expectations and don't communicate. An inflexible collaborator ("my way or the highway") is difficult to work with, but before you walk away, make sure that he or she is not correct. Some people are inflexible because they are correct. Differences in expectations usually arise about how much work will be done, who will do it, how fast it will be done, authorship, exclusivity of the collaboration, confidentiality of data, and future work. In the examples that follow, you will see how the same problems recur, and that the universal solution is diplomatic early clarification of everyone's expectations. What seems self-evident to you may not be so to others – communicate.

Examples of problems trainees or junior faculty have had with collaborators:
   Scenario 1: A postdoctoral fellow was asked to help recruit patients into a multi-center clinical trial. The fellow screened and recruited most of the

patients for the local study site and dealt with patient problems related to her specialty. The fellow was not included as an author in the eventual publication that included three investigators from each of ten sites.

Problem: The fellow expected authorship and did not get it. The faculty member and the fellow had different views about the importance of the fellow's contribution and the appropriate recognition.

Solution: When you collaborate, particularly with new collaborators, clarify everyone's expectations. In this case, it was too late and the fellow learnt a hard lesson.

Scenario 2: A senior faculty member asked a postdoctoral fellow who was working with another group to help a medical student with a project. The medical student had very little time for research and the fellow was spending a lot of time on the student's project rather than on his own work or projects for his group.

Problem: The fellow was doing work he expected the medical student to do; he expected to be an advisor and had become the laborer. The faculty member either had different expectations about the work load and who was going to do it or was not aware of the situation.

Solution: When you collaborate, particularly with new collaborators, clarify everyone's expectations. In this case, the fellow met with the faculty member and the medical student and diplomatically reset the boundaries.

Scenario 3: Two collaborating postdoctoral fellows were working in the same lab in the same general area and both proposed grant applications that, although not identical, were in the same broad area and used preliminary data they had both generated. When one of them approached their mentor about the problem, it emerged that the mentor had also submitted a grant on the topic with the same data.

Problem: Both fellows presumed they had exclusive rights to the lab's data and to a broad area of research. They also did not realize that their mentor had been planning a grant application in the same area.

Solution: Most research groups work in focused thematic areas, and collaborations between postdoctoral fellows provide synergy that enhances everyone's success. However, conflict can arise when trainees use each other's data, or data obtained collaboratively, for grant applications. Data generated by a particular laboratory are often used by everyone in the lab with attribution to the royal "we." For example, if your mentor has generated data that you are using in a grant you might write, "as we have previously shown…" Generally, the people whose data you include as part of your preliminary studies for a grant should be co-investigators or consultants. In other words, communicate with people and include them as collaborators and you will avoid some of these problems.

Scenario 4: Dr. B, a young faculty member, was asked to provide content expertise for a group reviewing the statistical methodology of papers related to a particular disease. He attended several meetings, read and categorized many papers about the disease, corrected the group's thinking about aspects of the disease, and made edits to drafts of the manuscript. Dr. B was not included as an author.

Problem: The writing group believed Dr. B was not a statistician and the content expertise was peripheral to the paper. Dr. B believed the review could not have been performed without his contribution and that he met the criteria for authorship.

Solution: When you collaborate, particularly with new collaborators, clarify everyone's expectations. Dr. B learnt two lessons – first, to clarify expectations early, and second, not to collaborate with this group again.

Scenario 5: Dr. C, a young faculty member, shared some unpublished data with Dr. D, a collaborator and established scientist. Dr. C was shocked to hear that Dr. D had shown these data in a talk at the national meeting. Although Dr. D had credited the data to her in the talk, Dr. C was annoyed because making these preliminary data public could enable competitors to scoop her and because her results could change with more experiments.

Problem: Dr. C had assumed that her data were shared in confidence. Dr. D had assumed that highlighting Dr. C's work in a talk was acceptable and even helpful.

Solution: If you share unpublished data, make sure you say if they are not for public distribution. Also, if you don't want slides copied or edited, send them as a pdf file.

Scenario 6: Dr. A and Dr. Z collaborated on a project and published a paper. Dr. Z was horrified to find that Dr. A had submitted a grant related to the project they had worked on collaboratively and had not included him as a collaborator. Even worse, Dr. A was now collaborating with one of Dr. Z's competitors.

Problem: Dr. Z had felt that future work on the topic, including grants, would be performed collaboratively. Dr. A felt that he did not need to include Dr. Z on every component of future work in the area and that he was free to expand his circle of collaborators and include anyone he wished.

Solution: It may seem self-evident to you that an area you have developed collaboratively should advance collaboratively. This may not be self-evident to your collaborators. Until you know and trust a collaborator, it is worth spelling out future plans. If you feel you have been treated badly, have a diplomatic discussion with your collaborator. If you cannot resolve the issue, one of two unsatisfactory outcomes is likely: either you will cease all collaboration and your erstwhile collaborator becomes a competitor, or you will continue to collaborate in limited areas for mutual advantage but do so cautiously, without sharing ideas.

Good academic citizenship

It is important to be a good academic citizen and to protect your time. Teaching, mentoring, serving on committees, giving talks, reviewing papers, reviewing grants, helping share the load for a sick colleague, interviewing prospective recruits, and having dinner with visiting faculty are all examples of activities that are important for the academic mission. A good mentor will protect you from excessive demands on your time early in your career. As your career develops and you take on more citizenship responsibilities, make sure that you choose commitments that will advance your career (Chapter 20), are compatible with your career trajectory, and do not impact your research adversely (Chapter 6).

Summary

1. Behave like a leader now, even if you are not sure you want to be a leader in the future.

2. Establish your career before you seek a leadership role.

3. A good collaborator shows up and is considerate.

4. Choose strong collaborators or collaborations.

4. Communication is the key to collaboration.

5. Be a good academic citizen but choose contributions that are compatible with your career trajectory and do not impact your research adversely.

Resources

1. What Got You Here Won't Get You There: How Successful People Become Even More Successful, by Marshall Goldsmith, Profile Books (2013).

2. The 21 Irrefutable Laws of Leadership: Follow Them and People Will Follow You, by John C Maxwell, Thomas Nelson (2007).

3. Vicens Q, Bourne PE. Ten simple rules for a successful collaboration. PLoS Comput Biol. 2007 Mar 30;3(3):e44. PMID: 17397252.

Chapter 27
Responsible conduct of research and conflict of interest

What is responsible conduct of research?

NIH defines responsible conduct of research (RCR) as the practice of scientific investigation with integrity. It involves the awareness and application of established professional norms and ethical principles in the performance of all activities related to scientific research. A simpler definition is doing the right thing. Scientists have responsibilities to other scientists, students, patients, animals, and society. Scientists, like everyone else, have competing interests, and it is important to reflect frequently on whether you are doing the right thing. NIH has identified nine RCR topics as particularly important (1), and I have copied those and used them as headers for each section below; we already discussed many of them earlier in the book.

1. Conflict of interest

It is difficult to define a conflict of interest. An Institute of Medicine report defined a conflict of interest as a set of circumstances that creates a risk that professional judgment or actions regarding a primary interest will be unduly influenced by a secondary interest (2). Few people believe that secondary interests influence their professional judgment or make them act differently, but the data indicate that we are all susceptible to bias (3). Moreover, it is important to realize that a conflict of interest exists even if you do not act in a biased way. It is the circumstances, rather than your actions, that place you in a situation where you have a conflict of interest. In fact, some argue that there are no "potential" or "perceived" conflicts of interest; if a reasonable person thinks there could be a conflict of interest, there is a conflict of interest (4). There are different types of conflict of interest; the most common are financial, scientific, and personal.

When do conflicts of interest apply: Conflicts of interest apply to every aspect of your professional life. You will be asked to declare conflicts of interest when you submit manuscripts, when you submit progress reports for grants, when you review grants, and when you give talks. You will be asked not to review papers or grants if you have a relevant conflict of interest. If you perform clinical research, conflicts of interest may apply to your research. For example, most institutions will not allow you to lead studies if you have a financial interest in the outcome (e.g., you discovered a drug that cured cancer in animals, patented it, and are now conducting the clinical trials).

Financial conflicts of interest: Financial conflicts of interest are the easiest to quantify, and most institutions require that faculty declare all conflicts that are greater than a certain amount, often $5,000 in a year. I declare all relevant financial conflicts of interest, even those less than $5,000, because I do not want to appear on the front page of the *New York Times* in an article titled: "Physician did not declare ties with drug company." Also, the amount of remuneration does not necessarily reflect the amount of potential bias. Physicians have a long history of unwittingly altering their behavior in response to free pizza, pens, and trinkets. Financial conflicts include remuneration for talks, consulting, expert opinion, directorships, stock ownership, gifts, patents (even though they may not have earned anything), and research support. If a drug company provides you with research support for a study, you must declare that as a conflict of interest even though technically the money is given to your institution.

Scientific conflicts of interest: Scientific conflicts of interest can arise if you are strongly invested in a particular intellectual position. For example, if you have made your reputation saying that salt does not cause hypertension, you may be perceived as biased if you review a paper saying the opposite. Scientific conflicts of interest can also arise if you are doing the same studies described in the work you are asked to review; however, working in the same area is not a conflict. Ask yourself – would a reasonable person think I could be biased?

Social conflicts of interest: Social conflicts of interest arise when your relationship with someone could be thought to influence your judgment. For this reason you will not review your mentees, mentors, colleagues at your institutions, collaborators, friends, relatives, and business partners. Friendly relationships are often obvious and public, but unfriendly ones are often private. If you dislike someone or feel rancor for something he or she did, don't be tempted to get payback. Rather, don't review the work.

Dealing with conflicts of interest: You can deal with conflicts of interest in three ways. First, you can avoid them by not entering a situation in which a conflict is relevant (e.g., avoid reviewing certain grants or papers). Second, you can manage them (e.g., if you are a patent holder for a drug, then independent researchers perform the clinical trials testing the drug). Third, you can declare them with the idea that transparency mitigates a conflict of interest by allowing people to view your actions or words through the lens of your conflict of interest. You will declare conflicts of interest in many situations. Make sure your declaration is accurate. It will be embarrassing if someone writes to complain that you have not declared a conflict of interest. This is not far-fetched because drug company payments to physicians are public knowledge and can be found on the *Dollars for Docs* site (5). If you give a talk, don't act ashamed of your conflict of interest slide and pass over it at lightning speed. Also, if you have several conflicts listed, don't joke: "I work with so many different companies I can't be biased." Rather, describe the relevance of any conflicts to your talk.

Keeping track of financial conflicts of interest: Keep a running log of your conflicts of interest so that you don't forget to list any when asked to do so (Chapter 21).

2. Policies regarding human subjects, live vertebrate animal subjects in research, and safe laboratory practices

Every institution requires ongoing training and certification for human, animal, and laboratory researchers. These policies safeguard the wellbeing of research subjects, animals, and people performing the research. It is important to keep your education and certification current and not to cheat in the on-line tests. Among the many principles that guide human research, two are worth emphasizing.

1) The consent form describes exactly what you will do – no more and no less. You cannot change a research protocol on the fly (except to protect the safety of a subject). For example, taking an extra tube of blood may seem trivial, but if you want an extra tube of blood you need to first amend the consent form and seek IRB approval.

2) A signed consent form does not mean you obtained informed consent. Handing subjects a consent form to sign does not mean they have provided informed consent. It is important to explain the study, the components of the consent form, and the risks and benefits of the study, and to solicit questions and check comprehension. It is also important to inform subjects that they can withdraw consent at any time and to record how you provided informed consent.

3. Mentor/mentee responsibilities and relationships

See Chapter 4.

4. Collaborative research, including collaborations with industry

Academic collaborations are discussed in Chapter 26. Collaborations with industry have different opportunities and challenges. In times past, medical researchers eschewed profit related to their research as being incompatible with professionalism. These days, medical researchers are encouraged to safeguard intellectual property, file patents, develop new therapies and devices, and start businesses. Moreover, researchers are encouraged to partner with industry in the search for additional funding sources. Collaborations with industry usually take one of six forms: 1) starting your own company; 2) partnering with industry and sharing ideas; 3) investigator-initiated research; 4) industry-initiated research; 5) consulting; and 6) continuing education.

1) Starting your own company: It is important to follow your institution's rules regarding companies that spring from findings made at the institution. Investigators generally establish their research careers and make some important, potentially marketable finding before starting a company. Therefore early career investigators do not usually start their own companies. If you are tempted, remember it is very difficult to run a company and an academic career successfully; usually one wins.

2) Partnering with industry and sharing ideas: A true partnership exists when each partner has unique skills and resources and shares these in pursuit of a common goal. Another type of partnership exists that is more akin to a venture capital investment. A company sees potential profit in what you are doing and provides funding for your studies in exchange for some guaranteed access to the intellectual property. Your institution's lawyers will spend a long time on a contract that specifies who gets what. Make sure you read the contract and stick to it. Such "private-public" partnerships face a fundamental challenge: the primary goals of academia are to serve science and patients, but the primary goal of a company is to serve its stockholders.

3) Investigator-initiated research: An investigator-initiated project is when you have an idea (usually related to a product a company makes) and receive support from the company (e.g., money, free drug, free assays) to test your idea. The company is not directly involved in the design, analysis, interpretation, or publication of the data. Again, there will be a contract that governs the arrangement between your institution and the company, particularly about the ownership of intellectual property that may derive from the studies. Also, the contract must allow you to publish the findings, no matter what they are.

4) Industry-initiated research: Industry-initiated research is when a company has a study it needs to perform (often a Phase III clinical trial) and asks investigators to participate. The company writes the protocol, collects data from the investigators, and oversees the interpretation and publication of the data. Investigators are paid, usually according to how many patients they recruit. Some academic investigators, often on the clinician-scholar/clinician-educator track, participate in many such industry-sponsored clinical trials.

5) Consulting: A company may ask for your opinion in an area it is working on and pay a fee for your time. Be careful that you are consulted for your expertise and not as a marketing ploy. Companies often seek to get "opinion leaders" on their side; one of the most effective ways to woo people is to socialize with them and also pay them.

6) Continuing education: Many universities prohibit faculty from attending continuing education functions hosted by companies and from speaking on their behalf. My impression is that individuals who serve on speakers' bureaus lose credibility in the eyes of their peers; don't give talks paid for by industry.

5. Peer review

See Chapter 10.

6. Data acquisition and laboratory tools; management, sharing and ownership

An important part of being a scientist is to keep meticulous records that show how data were generated and analyzed. The recent emphasis on sharing data means that others may reanalyze your data. Use appropriate statistical techniques and keep a record of the analysis pathway so that anyone can repeat it. Sharing data is important for science, but make sure you do not share data with subject identifiers and that you follow the policies of your institution. Many investigators believe that the data they have generated belong to them; in reality, at most places data belong to the institution. This can lead to disagreements and even legal battles when investigators leave and want to take "their" data with them.

7. Research misconduct and policies for handling misconduct

The most egregious cases of research misconduct have involved plagiarism (Chapter 8) and falsification or fabrication of data. These cases are only the tip of the iceberg. More common, and more difficult to identify, is cheating by selecting desirable data points and discarding others because "they must have been wrong," or repeating the same experiment 10 times until one gives a p-value <0.05. It is important to have a laboratory notebook that includes every data point from every experiment. Errors do indeed occur in experiments (e.g., you may have inadvertently forgotten to add the agonist). In such cases, annotate your notebook, explain your thinking, show the data to you supervisor and record the supervisor's comments in your notebook. It is important not to feel (nor to induce it in others) pressure to produce data compatible with a particular hypothesis. The data are the data (mentor Alastair Wood); hypotheses are often wrong no matter how smart or influential the people they emanated from. Journals have strict rules about the handling of figures and photographs (6) and you must adhere to these.

8. Responsible authorship and publication

We discussed responsibilities of authors and reviewers in Chapters 7 and 10.

9. The scientist as a responsible member of society, contemporary ethical issues in biomedical research, and the environmental and societal impacts of scientific research

Your responsibilities as a scientist extend into the community. It is important that you perform accurate and reproducible research and help society interpret you findings appropriately. If you are asked by the press to comment on one of your papers, you have a responsibility to do so, and to do so in a way that places the findings in appropriate context. We have all seen misleading news articles touting cures for cancer based on findings in cells or animal models.

Summary

1. Do the right thing.
2. Recognize that we all have conflicts of interest that can bias our judgment.
3. Keep track of your financial conflicts of interest.
4. Declare conflicts of interest when asked to do so.
5. Plagiarism and falsification and fabrication of data are the most egregious types of research misconduct but are only the tip of the iceberg.
6. The data are the data; your responsibility is to the data not the hypothesis.

Resources

1. NIH definition of responsible conduct of research.
   http://grants.nih.gov/grants/guide/notice-files/not-od-10-019.html
2. Institute of Medicine Conflict of Interest in Medical Research, Education, and Practice (April 21, 2009). http://www.iom.edu/Reports/2009/Conflict-of-Interest-in-Medical-Research-Education-and-Practice.aspx
3. Ariely, Dan The Honest Truth about Dishonesty, HarperCollins, 2012, p. 255, ISBN 978-0-06-218359-0, OCLC 757484553
4. McCoy MS, Emanuel EJ. Why there are no "potential" conflicts of interest. JAMA 2017;317:1721-2.
5. Dollars for Docs site. https://projects.propublica.org/docdollars/.
6. Rules about the handling of figures and photographs.
   http://www.aje.com/en/author-resources/articles/avoiding-image-fraud-7-rules-editing-images
6. American Association of Medical Colleges. The scientific basis of influence and reciprocity: A symposium.
   https://www.aamc.org/44826/search.html?q=influence&x=11&y=10
7. Ariely, Dan. Predictably Irrational: The Hidden Forces That Shape Our Decisions. Second edition in 2012., HarperCollins, 2008, ISBN 978-0-06-135323-9, OCLC 182521026
8. Ariely, Dan. The Upside of Irrationality: The Unexpected Benefits of Defying Logic at Work and at Home, HarperCollins, 2010, ISBN 978-0-06-199503-3, OCLC 464593990

Chapter 28

The seven (or so) deadly sins that hinder academic success

What is academic success?

Academic success does not mean the same thing to everyone. Different people place different value on the usual measures of success such as publishing a lot of papers, publishing in high-impact journals, getting tenure, building a productive research unit, having a lot of NIH funding, feeling fulfilled, performing meaningful research, being able balance family and work life, having the respect of your peers, being famous, winning prizes, helping patients, being a great clinician, teacher and scientist, and so on. You are the person who decides what academic success means, and you are the major determinant of that success. If a change in career track makes you more successful, it is success not failure.

The path to success is seldom a straight line

The careers of academic scientists and professional athletes are very similar. Both are extremely competitive and require innate talent, hard work, luck, good coaching, continuous improvement, a good team, discipline, focus, facing failure, and the ability to perform at the highest level consistently. Both careers are also unpredictable. This book may seem to imply that the path to academic success is a clearly mapped straight line – follow the map and you will get there. That is not the case. The path is seldom a straight line and yours may take you to unexpected places and through unexpected changes.

Can we predict academic success?

Is there a phenotype that predicts academic success? Sport is the best analogy. Potential top athletes need a high level of ability, but in that qualifying group it is difficult to predict individual success. You can deconstruct the skills a sport requires into components such as vertical leap, 50 yd time, reaction time, and so on. These measures have some predictive value, but the future performance of athletes with the same apparent skills differs substantially. Many highly ranked draft picks are not successful, and some undrafted athletes are very successful.

Just as in sport, you can quantify the individual attributes that are helpful for academic success, but a blend of attributes and how you apply them may be more important. Retrospectively, people usually attribute success to a combination of hard work, drive, initiative, talent, timing, and luck; but success is unpredictable. Nevertheless, there are some behaviors that predictably decrease the likelihood of success. This chapter summarizes the Dante's seven deadly sins (lust, pride, wrath, sloth, envy, greed, and gluttony) and others that affect academic success. I discussed many of the points in earlier chapters, and other writers have made many of the same observations (1,2).

Sins that hinder success

1. Lust (lack of)

It is hard to measure scientific lust, but you need it for success. The drive to do good science, love of the game, fire in the belly (mentor Grant Wilkinson) – call it what you want, is key. Drive is not enough; Pascal described four kinds of people: "zeal without knowledge; knowledge without zeal; neither knowledge nor zeal; both zeal and knowledge." You need both zeal and knowledge. But, remember no matter how zealous you are, at times the flame burns low in everyone. Science has ups and down – pace yourself and learn to deal with both adversity and success.

2. Pride

You will fail a lot. You will be rejected a lot. Your grants, papers, and ideas will all be rejected. You may never have failed an exam in your life, and now you may face failures that threaten your career. Failure feels devastating, but if you are too sensitive or too proud to cope effectively, an academic career will be impossible. Grow a thick skin quickly. Unfortunately, deafness to constructive feedback can be a byproduct of this thick skin. Retain a healthy perspective and the ability to listen.

3. Wrath

Angry at reviewers: Anger is the byproduct of pride. In other words, when you are rejected you feel that you are incontrovertibly right and the reviewer is wrong. Your anger may be justified, but it is not productive. For example, getting angry with a reviewer for being stupid, fussy, or careless is understandable but does not help. Rather, listen to the reviewer and channel your emotion into positive activity. Vent in private not in resubmissions or responses to reviewers.

Angry at people: There will always be differences of opinion between people. Opinions differ not only about scientific matters but also about performance, responsibilities, shared resources, attitudes, authorship, and so on. Recognizing a difference of opinion almost before it exists and resolving it is much easier than dealing with conflict. Anger and conflict affect relationships and productivity adversely. Learning to resolve disagreements and conflicts smoothly without anger is an important skill. Scientists have long memories – if you treat people badly they will never forget it. If you are diplomatic, there is seldom a need to make an enemy. If you make a mistake, apologize sincerely and make up for it.

4. Sloth

Successful scientists work very hard. Research is not a job that is "easier" than a clinical career. The hours are more flexible, but most successful researchers put in a lot of hours. Putting the hours in is not enough; efficiency and appropriate allocation of time are just as important (Chapter 6).

5. Envy

There will always be scientists who have more papers, bigger labs, more postdocs, higher salaries, and more titles than you do. Envy is anger at yourself for not being more successful and at others for being too successful. It is not helpful. Be aware of your own career trajectory and focus on that. As Mr. Hawke writes in *Rules for a Knight*, a book that has many teachings relevant to an academic career, (3) "there are only two possible outcomes whenever you compare yourself to another, vanity or bitterness, and both are without value." Comparing yourself to others can also make you feel inferior even though you might have achieved a lot. If you feel useless remind yourself of what you have achieved.

6. Greed

Other people's careers are also important; you should apportion credit for work fairly. The benefits of being selfish, climbing on the heads of others, and taking advantage of people are short-lived. If you get a reputation for being greedy, you will find fewer and fewer people willing to collaborate with you.

7. Gluttony

Don't overload your plate. You need research time to do research. Beware of slipping into cognitive dissonance – *I am aiming at the physician-scientist tenure track, a K award, and then an RO1. I do 3 clinics a week, serve on the IRB committee, direct a teaching course, and cover the wards for 4 months a year.*

8. Low curiosity

Scientists have a lot of curiosity. They ask questions and want to know why and how something happens. Most good scientists I know could easily be studying something completely different with just as much enthusiasm. A medical training on the other hand discourages curiosity because we are taught there is only one correct answer to a clinical problem. You have to have outstanding questions for a successful career in science, and you discover these through curiosity.

9. Low creativity

Good questions are the foundation of scientific creativity. We have all read papers in high-impact journals where the authors took information available to all of us and asked a question that is brilliant but (in hindsight) obvious. Why did we not make the same connections and see the same question? Can one cultivate creativity? Creativity springs from knowing a lot, defining a question, looking for approaches or solutions others have developed (often in areas unrelated to yours), and then making unexpected connections. The enemy of creativity is being wedded to one idea or technique – a person with a hammer can find a lot of nails. Learning to develop and select those ideas that are new, important, interesting, feasible, and testable is a big part of your research training. Keep a file of potential ideas – memory is short. Take a fresh look at your old ideas from time to time. Think hard before you dive into a new project (Chapter 3).

10. Not reading and writing at lot

Read, Read, Read: Reading is how we learn and how we get ideas. Read in your area, read around your area, and read where your curiosity takes you. If you do not know the literature surrounding your research project much better than your mentor does, you have not read enough. Learn how to read effectively – sometimes for breadth, and sometimes for depth. Scan the contents page of selected journals regularly. My list has some general high-quality journals (*Science, Nature, Nature Medicine, Journal of Clinical Investigation, New England Journal of Medicine, Lancet, Annals of Internal Medicine, Science Translational Medicine*) and then some specific to my research or clinical work (*Hypertension, Clinical Pharmacology and Therapeutics, Nature Genetics, Circulation,* and several rheumatology journals). Make your own list. Many journals will automatically email you the contents page of each new issue. I find it helpful to set aside a regular time to scan journals and to read; I often scan journals for articles on Friday afternoon, print some of them, and read them over the weekend.

Write, Write, Write: The ability to write adequately is not an inborn talent. It can be learnt. Writing is slow, hard work and requires practice and attention to detail. The only way to publish papers or to receive grants is to write.

11. No perseverance

You will be rejected often and many experiments won't work. Persevere. Although perseverance is essential, persevering in the wrong direction or with a flawed approach is not a good idea – use your mentors for guidance.

12. Ignorance

To succeed you need not only knowledge but tools. Doing research is not instinctive. You cannot expect to be successful in research without training, just as you would not expect to be a successful surgeon without training. A medical training has almost nothing to do with research. Decide how you will get the scientific skills you need. Will it be through apprenticeship and working closely with a successful mentor, or will it include a degree such as a PhD, MSCI or

MPH? Learning to do research is like learning a new language – it is hard, it takes time, and it is easier if you are fully immersed in it and have experts to coach you.

13. Poor environment
Be careful where you build your research house. A supportive environment helps grow your career. This environment includes things like a mentor, collaborators, space, protected time, salary support, startup money, research facilities, the culture of the institution, a critical mass of researchers, and administrative support. If you have been successful in one environment, moving to a new environment when you are starting an independent career can be dangerous unless you are following or joining a strong mentor.

14. No mentor
Having no mentor, or an inappropriate mentor, is a great disadvantage (Chapter 2).

15. No mentoring committee
Not having a mentoring committee or not using the committee is handicapping yourself (Chapter 5).

16. Inability to listen
You will get lots of advice and criticism – solicited and unsolicited. There is a skill to hearing an opinion, processing and evaluating it, and finally acting. Some people become so argumentative and defensive in the face of constructive criticism that they do not hear the suggestions. Others think they have heard the suggestions but misinterpret their significance. Advisors often speak in a "code" of understated opinions, and unless you are listening, it is easy to miss what they are really communicating (Chapter 4).

17. Lack of focus
Focus your career story: It is important that you become expert in one area. As a "name" in an area it will be easier for you to publish your papers and get your grants funded because reviewers acknowledge your background expertise. The publications on your CV tell the story of your career focus.

Focus your grants: Focus your aims and experiments so that the questions are clear and there is a logical flow and you are not "all over the place."

Focus your work: Think about goals and deliverable units (i.e., papers). A large mass of "cool" preliminary data that are never published will only buy you credibility for so long – at some stage you have to deliver.

Focus your collaborations: Choose high quality collaborators whose work advances yours and *vice versa*.

Focus does not mean doing the same thing forever: It is almost certain that 10 years from now you will be doing very different work. This occurs by differentiating and diversifying into new areas – usually in a way that is driven by the results of your past and current science. There can be a tension between diversifying your research portfolio and maintaining focus. Appropriate diversification almost always has a logical narrative within the context of your career path and this narrative is easily visible on your CV. Different projects that are related in some way provide synergy to each other. On the other hand, a constellation of "cool" unrelated projects suggest poor focus.

18. No funding

At some stage in your academic career you will have to get funding to progress. The only way to get funding is to apply for funding. Maximize your chances by learning how to write grants, by submitting the same grant to different places (within the rules of each organization), and by having colleagues review your grants before you submit them. Keep trying. Look at successful grants and learn from them. Listen to reviewers. Take grant writing courses.

19. Rush to independence

It is important to become independent, but not at the risk of crashing your career. Continued collaboration with your mentor has many advantages; however, you may not look independent. Generally, this apparent lack of independence can be debunked in letters of support for grants or promotion packages, or in the personal statement section of biosketches. A complete break from your mentor can be disastrous (Chapter 4).

20. Not keeping track

It is important to keep track of your career in different ways so that you can take action early to avoid problems, particularly as regards funding or promotion. Updating your CV regularly will help you keep track of important areas: 1) scientific productivity; 2) funding; and 3) scientific reputation – the three major criteria for promotion on the tenure track (Chapters 20 and 21). Keep track of ideas for grants; write them down and keep them in a folder. Keep track of when your funding will run out so that you can plan well ahead of time.

21. Poor planning

It is easier to avoid a mess than to get out of it; this is the point of planning. Running a research operation is like running a small business and instead of widgets we produce papers and grants (mentor Alastair Wood). You will need to learn to manage operations, people, and money, as well as your science. Set goals and deadlines for yourself and others. The pipeline for your funding and productivity requires both short-term and long-term planning

22. Negativity

Everyone has self-doubt and negative thoughts, but these can become all-consuming and self-fulfilling – sometimes termed the "imposter syndrome."

Cultivate confidence under fire and positive energy. Don't become known as a glass-is-half-empty person. Why should your mentors believe in you if you don't believe in yourself? As Mr. Hawke writes, "Be enthusiastic or be gone!" (3).

23. Passivity

Things won't happen unless you make them happen. Hope is not a plan (attribution unclear – Rick Page used it as a title for a book in 2003). Do not expect your mentor to be responsible for your success. Direct your research, your networking, your interests, your scientific relationships, your grant applications, and your career. Feeling entitled (even subconsciously) is dangerous; things won't just happen.

24. Research misconduct

Plagiarism, fabrication, and fraud are at the extremes of scientific misconduct. More common and subtle is unacceptable behavior in gray areas. Doing the right thing is the credo of scientific research (Chapter 27).

25. Poor resilience

Resilience, the ability to bounce back from failure, is an important skill. After a failure, mourn briefly if you need to, but learn and move on to the next battle with confidence. Your favorite sports team does not win every match but strives to play harder and better after a loss. Several techniques can help you with resilience: don't take things personally, be optimistic, recall your past successes, think about the success of people around you, see the positive side of your struggles, remember that many people are worse off than you, and get support from others (4).

Summary

Some early warning signs:
1. No clear hypothesis.
2. No clear mentor or mentor is disengaged.
3. No grant submissions.
4. Publication record is poor.
5. Conflict.
6. No mentoring committee or it has not met.
7. No one else looked at grant before submission.
8. Too much clinical time.
9. Poor focus.
10. Recently moved to a new institution.
11. The future path is unclear.

Some tips for success:
1. Have good mentors and a committee.
2. Study important questions.
3. Work hard with good people.
4. Learn skills.
5. Read widely.
6. Write.
7. Have a research portfolio.
8. Ride the punches.
9. Develop independence at the right speed.
10. Be aware (where your career is; what advisors are saying to you).
11. Compensate for weaknesses.

Resources

1. Lee SJ. Tips for success as an academic clinical investigator. J Clin Oncol 2013;6:811-13.

2. Kohan DE. Moving from trainee to junior faculty: a brief guide. Physiologist 2014;57:3-6. PMID: 24605413.

3. Hawke, E. Rules for a Knight. Knopf. First Edition (November 10, 2015) ISBN-10: 0307962334.

4. Parker-Pope, Tara. How to build resilience in mid-life. New York Times, July 25, 2017.

Abbreviations, acronyms, jargon, and slang

(See Glossary of NIH terms http://grants.nih.gov/grants/glossary.htm#R)

CDA: VA Career Development Award.

CE and CS: Clinician-educator and clinician-scholar tracks (often used interchangeably).

CRC: Clinical Research Center.

CSR: Center for Scientific Review; handles NIH grant submissions and reviews.

CTSA: Clinical and Translational Science Award.

CV: Curriculum Vitae.

DOD: Department of Defense.

eRA Commons: NIH web portal for grant submissions and reviews.

ESI: Early stage investigator; a New Investigator (no previous substantive NIH support as PI) who is within 10 years of completing a terminal research degree or completing medical residency.

F32: Mentored training grant to an individual.

IACUC: Institutional Animal Care and Use Committee.

IAR: Internet assisted review section of NIH eRA Commons.

ICs: Institutes and Centers (NIH).

ICMJE: International Committee of Medical Journal Editors.

IDP: Individual Development Plan.

IRB: Institutional Review Board.

JIT: Just-in-time information requested by NIH for grants.

KO1: Mentored research grant for individuals with a clinical or non-clinical doctoral degree; most often PhDs doing basic research.

KO8: Mentored research grant for individuals with a clinical doctoral degree (e.g., MD, Pharm D, DO) doing basic research.

K23: Mentored research grant for individuals with a clinical doctoral degree (e.g., MD, Pharm D, DO) doing patient oriented research.

K99/R00: The "Pathway to Independence Award" is aimed at individuals is a hybrid combining 1-2 years of mentored K-type funding with 3 years of independent R-type funding. It is open to non-U.S. citizens.

Merit Awards: VA research grant similar to an RO1.

NCE: No-cost extension.

NCI: National Cancer Institute.

NHLBI: National Heart, Lung, and Blood Institute.

NIGMS: National Institute of General Medical Sciences.

NIH: National Institutes of Health.

NIH RePORTER: A searchable website of NIH grants and grantees.

NOA or NOGA: Notice of grant award (official notification of funding).

Other support: Active and pending grant support.

PA: Program announcement; invites grant applications in an area. No funds set aside.

Payline: The percentile up to which grants are funded.

PI: Principal Investigator.

Pink sheets: Summary statement (reviews of your grant).

PMC: PubMed Central. A repository of full-text scientific publications.

PMCID: PubMed Central ID number.

PMID: PubMed ID number.

PO: Program Official (or Program Officer); fosters an IC's science, advises applicants.

PO1 and PPG: A multi-investigator multi-project grant; Program Project Grant.

RFA: Request for applications; requests grant applications in an area. Sometimes recur. Funds set aside.

RFP: Request for proposals; requests applications for a contract to perform a particular task. Often does not recur. Funds set aside.

R01: The bread-and-butter NIH research grant used by all ICs.

R21: A 2 year grant for exploratory research; total direct costs cannot exceed $275,000.

R03: A grant for small limited project; usually limited to 2 years with direct costs of $50,000 per year.

SRO: Scientific review officer; arranges study sections.

Streamlined: A euphemism for a grant that is triaged or not discussed.

Summary statement: The official reviews of your grant.

T32: Also known as Ruth L. Kirchstein awards; mentored training grants.

VA: Veterans Administration.

Index

www.ingramcontent.com/pod-product-compliance
Lightning Source LLC
Chambersburg PA
CBHW081718220526
45468CB00008B/1887